Sleep Better with
Natural Therapies

of related interest

Breaking Free from Persistent Fatigue
Lucie Montpetit
ISBN 9781848191013
eISBN 9780857010810

Make Yourself Better
A Practical Guide to Restoring Your Body's
Wellbeing through Ancient Medicine
Philip Weeks
ISBN 9781848190122
eISBN 9780857010773

The Mystery of Pain
Douglas Nelson
ISBN 9781848191525
eISBN 9780857011169

Principles of NLP
What It Is, How It Works, and What It Can Do for You
Joseph O'Connor and Ian McDermott
Foreword by Robert Dilts
ISBN 9781848191617
eISBN 9780857011367
Part of the Discovering Holistic Health series

Principles of Hypnotherapy
What It Is, How It Works, and What It Can Do for You
Vera Peiffer
ISBN 9781848191266
eISBN 9780857011022
Part of the Discovering Holistic Health Series

Sleep Better with Natural Therapies

A Comprehensive Guide to Overcoming Insomnia, Moving Sleep Cycles and Preventing Jet Lag

Peter Smith

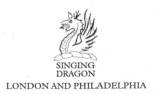

SINGING
DRAGON
LONDON AND PHILADELPHIA

Disclaimer

Every effort has been made to ensure that the information contained in this book is correct, but it should not in any way be substituted for medical advice. Readers should always consult a qualified medical practitioner before incorporating any of the therapies or supplements mentioned in this book into their treatment plan. Neither the author nor the publisher takes any responsibility for any consequences of any decision made as a result of the information contained in this book.

First published in 2014
by Singin Dragon
73 Collier Street
London N1 9BE, UK
and
400 Market Street, Suite 400
Philadelphia, PA 19106, USA

www.singingdragon.com

Front cover image source: iStockphoto®. The cover image is for illustrative purposes only, and any person featuring is a model.

Library of Congress Cataloging in Publication Data
Smith, Peter K.
  Sleep better with natural therapies : a holistic guide to
overcoming insomnia and restoring a healthy
sleep cycle / Peter Smith.
    pages cm
  Includes bibliographical references and index.
  ISBN 978-1-84819-182-2 (alk. paper)
  1. Insomnia--Alternative treatment. 2. Sleep disorders--Alternative treatment. I. Title.
  RC548.S65 2014
  616.8'4982--dc23
                              2013016024

British Library Cataloguing in Publication Data
A CIP catalogue record for this book is available from the British Library

ISBN 978 1 84819 182 2
eISBN 978 0 85701 140 4

Printed and bound in Great Britain by Bell & Bain Ltd, Glasgow

Contents

Preface

The insomnia cure programme in this book started with the already tried and tested cognitive behavioural therapy (CBT) insomnia programme developed at the Harvard Medical School as a foundation and then added both physical and psychological techniques to make it even more powerful and effective at overcoming insomnia.

The key additions include:

- An innovative technique called virtual darkness that enables you to adjust the timing of the release of the sleep hormone melatonin in the evening and the use of total darkness in your bedroom which maximises and maintains melatonin production production throughout the night.

- The use of bright light therapy in the morning further coordinates melatonin production. The addition of specific supplements to this bright light therapy technique increases the speed of melatonin production, which in turn intensifies the natural pressure which should force us to fall asleep, and yet other supplements assist the bright light therapy in coordinating the activity of our internal biological clock which is at the heart of our 24 hour sleep–wake cycles.

- Additional supplements increase the natural production of the sedating neurotransmitters (brain chemicals) serotonin and gamma-aminobutyric acid (GABA) which improve sleep and tranquillise the mind.

• Even with all of the above, the stress hormone cortisol can put a spanner in the works and prevent you from being able to fall asleep when its levels do not decline in the evening as they should. Elevated evening cortisol is a product of internal stress responses; these may be too subtle for you to even know they're happening. On the insomnia programme in this book you will undergo an intensive retraining of your autonomic nervous system to teach your nervous system a new ability that will permanently eliminate the problem of elevated evening cortisol interfering with your sleep. This relaxation response training is included in the original CBT insomnia programme but is underutilised and not always completed adequately. I have extensively added to and expanded this important technique, drawing from the latest understandings of how we produce stress responses and what we can do to ensure that your brain will allow cortisol levels to fall in the evening.

• Cognitive hypnotherapy exercises have been added to enhance the behavioural techniques in reprogramming the subconscious mind. During each step of the insomnia curing programme you will use specific mental exercises and listen to different self-hypnosis recordings to cover multiple problems causing insomnia.

How to Use this Book

There are two sections in this book: one on how to treat insomnia and become a good sleeper and the other on how to control and move your sleep cycles (i.e. the timing of when you wake up, switch on, switch off and fall asleep). You may want to go straight to the treatment section for your problem, especially if you have insomnia, however insomnia and sleep cycle disorders have some things in common that you need to know to understand the treatments. Those common aspects are discussed in this section so they are not repeated later on. For example, I will show you how to change your natural melatonin (the sleep hormone) production to treat both insomnia and move sleep cycles, therefore what you need to know about melatonin to use this book is described in this section. Whichever part of the book you're interested in, even if it's just jet lag, read this chapter first before branching off.

I'm aware that people with insomnia especially may be desperate to get started as soon as possible to overcome the insomnia and to address the urgency of your problem there are a few things you can start doing straight away, from today. You can begin changing the duration of the stress responses your brain and nervous system makes by developing the ability to switch on a parasympathetic relaxation response in your system. This will start to eliminate the influence of the anti-sleep (wake-up) hormone called cortisol; it takes several weeks for this to produce a pronounced effect, so the sooner you start the better. You'll learn all about how your stress responses work in Step 2 of the insomnia programme, but for now all you need to do is switch on a parasympathetic relaxation response for about 25 minutes once a day.

Also, in about four weeks you will need to have completed the sleep diary you'll find in Step 1 of the insomnia cure, so you can start making your sleep diary within the next few days. It's often quite revealing to find out how much sleep you are or are not actually getting. Along with reading this book I hope that these two exercises give your mind a feeling that it is already beginning to do something.

You may also need to decrease evening cortisol if you are a night owl (i.e. have a delayed sleep cycle) so you should also opt to start a parasympathetic relaxation response straight away.

Written instructions on the parasympathetic relaxation response are available on my websites or you can be guided through the technique with a free recording available via e-mail. To receive the digital recordings to accompany this book, simply send me an e-mail asking for the sleep better recordings; my address is sleep@the-sleep-solution.com. This recording is specifically designed to be the first step of your insomnia treatment and includes visualisation exercises for your subconscious mind to see yourself becoming a good sleeper in the future. If the quality and quantity of your sleep is adequate and your interest here is only in moving the timing of your sleep ask for Parasympathetic Relaxation Response Recording, which is a generic recording without any special insomnia exercises. See Contact Details and Getting the Free Recordings at the end of the book for my website addresses.

PART 1

Understanding Sleep

～ 1.1 ～

What Makes Us Sleep and Wake?

This book is meant to be a simple to follow, practical how-to self-help manual for people with sleep problems; it is not meant to be an academic reference book on sleep medicine and sleep science. However, some scientific explanation is necessary in this self-help book for you to understand how you are going to treat and change the systems in your body, brain and mind that control your sleep. I had real patients on the one hand telling me they wanted the book to be as simple a self-help manual as possible and students and colleagues on the other wanting an academic book on sleep, but this book is primarily written to equip people with the self-help tools they need to sleep better, as today the academic reader can quickly look up further research material on all the remedies and techniques used in this book. If you're a non-science person don't be put off by the long words used in this introductory chapter – you don't have to memorise any of it, just read through it and understand the following points:

- You have a biological clock in your brain that times the release of hormones that affect when you wake up and fall asleep.

- The biological clock is reset by bright light, specifically blue wavelengths of light in the morning.

- Too much light, specifically blue wavelengths of light in the evening, delays and reduces the production of the hormone melatonin which plays a central role in making you fall asleep.

- We can deliberately reset our biological clock to sleep better and move the timing of when we fall asleep and wake up (our sleep–wake cycle) by using bright (blue) light treatment.

- We can increase both the *amount* of melatonin we produce and move the peak production *time* by eliminating blue light in the evening and night.

- A chemical called adenosine builds up in our bodies throughout the day which sedates the brain, making us feel sleepy. We can increase the build-up of adenosine by increasing our level of physical activity and exercise.

- Sometime before we fall asleep our internal body temperature starts to drop and shut down our internal activity levels; this signals to our system when it's time to sleep. Prior to bedtime we must allow our body to lose heat and cool down; we can even trick our body into feeling sleepier by deliberately warming ourselves up then quickly cooling ourselves down.

What makes us sleep

Exactly how and why we sleep is not completely understood despite considerable scientific research, and there is more to how and why we sleep than discussed in this chapter, but those things are of no use to us because I don't know how to change or influence them. Everything in this chapter is included for a practical purpose because these are the things that control our sleep that we can control and influence ourselves.

Adenosine makes us sleep

You'll find many sources discussing melatonin as though it's the only sleep-inducing compound in the body, however there is another chemical that makes us sleep called *adenosine*.

In the brain adenosine acts as an inhibitory neurotransmitter that suppresses arousal. It continuously builds up in the blood every hour you are awake and after 16–18 hours awake the adenosine level creates drowsiness and increasing difficulty in staying awake; this is called *sleep pressure* and should eventually force us to sleep. While we sleep adenosine is broken down and removed from the body and after enough quality sleep adenosine levels are sufficiently low for us to wake up feeling wide awake and refreshed. It is believed that when we do not get enough sleep (quantity and quality count) the adenosine levels are not adequately lowered and the 'leftover' adenosine makes us feel drowsy the next day; this is called *sleep debt*. Indications that you have a sleep debt are yawning, heavy eyelids, difficulty concentrating, feeling tired and a desire to sleep.

When a person does not sleep for a long time (several days) the levels of adenosine will interfere with the brain's ability to stay awake so significantly it can force people into micro-sleeps even while standing up or driving. Eventually the high levels of adenosine will incapacitate the brain and people will fall into a deep sleep even in the presence of outside noise and disturbances; this phenomenon has been observed in soldiers during protracted battles, for example.

Caffeine blocks the sites in the brain where adenosine exerts its influence; it does not, however, break down adenosine or stop it being made, so tea and coffee can only temporarily offset sleep debt. Tea and coffee can also have other stimulating effects by increasing dopamine.

I do not know of any effective natural remedies to influence adenosine levels that might help cure insomnia, except for one thing. Adenosine levels build up as a by-product of us burning up (or metabolising) energy. Have you ever had the experience of falling asleep easily then sleeping deeply like a log after a *physically* exhausting day? It is believed that increasing our energy turnover with physical activity/exercise increases adenosine levels, which in turn builds up a stronger sleep pressure. If you're having trouble falling asleep try doing a lot of exercise, it's good for you anyway.

Under normal circumstances, after say 17 hours awake, the pressure to sleep exerted by adenosine is not overwhelming on its own and works together with the assistance of a second sleep compound, the sleep hormone melatonin.

Melatonin makes us sleep

You've probably already heard of melatonin, it's a hormone produced in our pineal gland after dark that makes us feel sleepy and sleep deeply. Melatonin is also a very powerful naturally produced antioxidant involved in repairing and protecting brain and body from free radical damage and ageing. It is believed that melatonin has powerful anti-cancer effects and a lack of melatonin is associated with an increased risk of cancer, particularly of the breast and prostate (see www.sleep-solution.com for more on the positive health effects of melatonin).

The way it is supposed to work is when light stops entering the eyes the body senses the sun has gone down and the night has begun it releases melatonin from the pineal gland, the production of melatonin starts to soar, eventually hitting us with a wave of sleepiness. A simple way to think about it is that light entering the eyes puts a clamp on the pineal gland stopping melatonin production; after dark when light stops entering the eyes the clamp is removed and the pineal gland releases melatonin. We will see later that not all wavelengths of light have the same effect and it is only bluish light that stops melatonin production. In the morning, light entering the eyes reapplies the clamp to the pineal gland and melatonin production stops again.

Incidentally in extreme conditions (usually experimental) when people and or animals live in complete darkness and in some totally blind people when absolutely no light signals reach the brain at all melatonin will still be produced on a regular scheduled basis under the control of the biological clock located in the brain. The biological clock does not keep perfect 24-hour time, however, and without the benefit of external bright light signals resetting the timing of the clock the schedule gradually drifts out of sync with the outside world. We will look at the biological clock and how to take control of it to help our sleep later.

Melatonin is like your brain's own naturally produced sleeping drug and in this book you will learn how to coax every last drop of melatonin out of your pineal gland to induce good quality sleep every night and benefit from melatonin's powerful anti-ageing and anti-cancer properties.

Melatonin is synthesised from serotonin (the neurotransmitter believed to be involved in depression) which in turn is made from the amino acid tryptophan.

L-Tryptophan → Serotonin → Melatonin

Serotonin concentrations are higher in the pineal gland than in any other part of the body and the levels of serotonin in the pineal gland fall by more than 80 per cent soon after the onset of darkness, as it is converted into melatonin. Supplementing tryptophan last thing at night feeds the brain the primary building block it uses to make serotonin and melatonin. Interestingly it appears that supplementing tryptophan has other sleep-enhancing effects in addition to facilitating the production of melatonin.

Melatonin levels should ideally rise quite rapidly in the evening and hit you with an intense sensation of sleepiness. In some people, however, melatonin levels rise too slowly to create a sufficiently intense sensation of sleepiness to send them to sleep and it's all too easy for these people to simply override, ignore or miss the weak signal of tiredness they experience. The cause of a slow melatonin release could be excess artificial light in the evening or simply individual biology, or a combination of the two.

The good news is we can increase the rate at which melatonin levels rise in the evening to help us fall asleep with a combination of bright light therapy (from a bright blue light therapy device) first thing in the morning and a high healthy dose of vitamin B-12. An additional benefit we gain from this treatment is it also speeds up the rate at which melatonin levels *fall in the morning* helping us to wake up more quickly. This combination of vitamin B-12 and bright light treatment is one of the unique protocols I use to treat sleep problems.

Melatonin can be bought as a supplement and has become quite popular. You can complete the insomnia treatment in this book with or without supplementing extra melatonin. You can just use the techniques discussed in this book to increase your natural melatonin production or if you want to you can supplement additional melatonin as an alternative sleeping pill. If you are currently taking sleeping pills my advice is to use melatonin supplements as a transitional stepping stone to help you come off the sleeping pills. I will discuss this in Step 5 of the Insomnia Cure Step-by-Step Treatment Programme.

Back in the 1990s I debated for a long time over the safety of artificially supplementing this powerful hormone. There are no proven negative health effects associated with taking melatonin and the consensus of opinion is that melatonin is both a safe and beneficial antioxidant, protecting the brain from ageing and perhaps reducing brain and breast cancer risk. It is not available for sale in the UK, but it is completely legal to buy it from overseas for personal use. I buy mine from iherb.com.

When I compared the risks of melatonin, which have been shown to be minimal and mainly hypothetical, with the positive health benefits of melatonin, which have been shown to be considerable, I decided that I would use it personally and recommend it in my practice. When one also takes into account the effects of lack of sleep melatonin comes out looking very good; I've been looking for 15 years for evidence that melatonin is not safe, but so far none has emerged.

You can find numerous blogs about melatonin giving people nightmares and feeling drowsy. I myself get nightmares when I take above 2–3 mg of melatonin, so if you have this problem try a lower dose or maybe melatonin is not for you, but it's not a *serious* medical side-effect. As for drowsiness, isn't that kind of the whole point to taking melatonin! It's like sleeping pills – you're supposed to feel drowsy and absolutely should not be driving a car or doing anything similar; the issue is timing. By adjusting the dose you shouldn't feel drowsy the next day at all, but rather you should feel refreshed having had a good night's sleep.

On the positive side studies on middle-aged rats given supplemental night-time melatonin resulted in the rats living longer. The gains in life expectancy were quite considerable in some cases, the equivalent of an increase of 12 human years! Someone tried to put me off melatonin by showing me a study that found that although the rats did live longer and remain healthier during those extra years, in the end they declined in health and died more rapidly than the un-medicated rats. I don't know about you but that sounds ideal! To gain some extra years and be healthy up to the end, then rapidly check out, sounds better than the drawn out slow decline many people experience.

If you have bipolar syndrome and are having trouble sleeping you *must* do whatever you have to make yourself sleep. In this context melatonin can be very useful and you should learn how to use it (dosage, etc.), so you have it ready and available to you if you ever need it.

Compared with sleeping pills melatonin does not cause significant dependency or morning drowsiness when used at the right dosage. In fact, as just mentioned, far from drowsy you should feel refreshed the next morning.

Despite its potential usefulness melatonin can be tricky to get to work properly and may require considerable experimentation to establish the dosage and timing that suits you. See the discussion in Appendix 4 to help you to choose and use the right melatonin for you.

Melatonin and adenosine are not the only important chemicals controlling our sleep–wake cycles that we can influence; another key player that we must understand is the stress hormone cortisol.

Evening cortisol prevents us from sleeping

Cortisol levels should rise in the morning wakening us up then fall, stepping out of the way by the evening to allow us to fall asleep. Hidden internal stress responses can prevent this from happening.

It's become popular to think of cortisol in a negative light. Search online and cortisol is blamed for weight gain especially belly fat, weak immunity, heart disease and more; the impression you get is that cortisol is all bad. What you may not know is that, like melatonin, cortisol levels should rise and fall on a 24-hour cycle. Cortisol is one of our fight or flight stress hormones, it causes the release of glucose and fatty acids from the liver into the blood stream which gives our brain and muscles fuel for energy production. In the morning shortly after melatonin levels fall we should get a surge in cortisol levels which is intended to wake us up, activate the immune system, make us mentally alert and active during the day. As the day wears on cortisol levels should decline so that by the evening the energy and alertness that cortisol gives us should be gone and have fizzled out leaving the way clear, so to speak, for adenosine and melatonin to send you to sleep. In Figure 1.1, Healthy cortisol cycles, you can see how cortisol surges in the morning then drops to its minimum level by early evening essentially stepping out the way for the melatonin to begin to exerting its effects. In the morning melatonin drops out of the way allowing us to wake up and the cortisol to give us a surge of energy and peak performance.

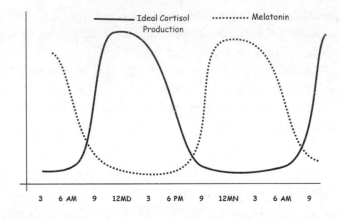

Figure 1.1: Healthy cortisol cycles

For many people, however, this does not happen and cortisol levels remain high throughout the day and, more importantly, into the evening because their internal physiology and psychology over-produce stress responses which maintain an elevated level of cortisol production. Chronic unhealthy stress responses cause cortisol to remain high in the evening. Notice also how the levels flatten out over 24 hours compared to the ideal big rise and fall throughout the day seen with healthy cortisol cycles. The levels also fluctuate frequently due to repeated stress responses. If this situation persists for long enough the adrenal glands can become fatigued and unable to even 'muster up' a healthy morning surge of cortisol. See Figure 1.2, Unhealthy stress responses and cortisol production.

Stress responses can occur in the background; you may not notice them or feel stressed, however, your internal physiology may be maintaining an elevated level of activity and cortisol that interferes with your ability to fall asleep. We can use our understanding of what triggers stress responses to eliminate the triggers which produce them from our evening environment. Just simply watching sports and thrillers on the TV, for example, has been shown to produce stress responses and elevate cortisol if they are exciting and entertaining. While you are training your body to become a good sleeper you need avoid any stimuli that can provoke evening stress responses for several hours before bed.

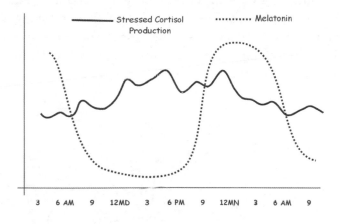

Figure 1.2: Unhealthy stress responses and cortisol production

Another thing we can do is teach our nervous system how to switch off stress responses quickly and efficiently to allow our cortisol levels to naturally decline as they should. On the insomnia cure in this book you do a long intensive relaxation training programme that I have found to be the only reliable way to permanently eliminate the problem of excess cortisol inhibiting sleep. By completing this training programme you will teach your brain and nervous system how to quickly drop into a deeply relaxed state and switch off all pre-existing stress responses. This technique will not stop your nervous system from producing stress responses in the first place, but it will equip your nervous system with the new skill of being able to switch off stress responses within 30 minutes or less as opposed to having them lingering on in the background for hours on end. In Figure 1.3, Cortisol cycles after relaxation training, you can see the type of improvement in the 24-hour cortisol cycle you could expect within three months of training. Although the person still has a nervous system that routinely over-produces stress responses elevating background cortisol levels they now have the ability to switch off the stress responses and allow cortisol levels to fall. This should significantly improve their health in a number of ways, including increased immunity, because constant elevated cortisol levels are taxing and depleting the immune system. More significantly for our purposes here the relaxation training will enable your system to lower cortisol levels in the evening enabling you to sleep better.

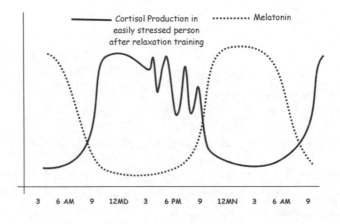

Figure 1.3: Cortisol cycles after relaxation training

The purpose of this book is to get you sleeping better and the relaxation training programme should be sufficient to remove the problem of evening cortisol for most people, however it is possible to change your internal stress responses further so that you produce less in the first place by remodelling and reprogramming stressful, traumatic and painful memories using neurolinguistic programming (NLP) and cognitive hypnotherapy techniques. This is not something you can do at home by yourself and requires the assistance of a practitioner. For most people this is an optional extra, however there are a few people who have such a highly strung disposition or who carry such a lot of emotional stresses that they are unable to successfully perform the relaxation training and have no choice but to work on their internal emotional stresses first if they want to prevent inappropriate stress responses interfering with their health and ability to sleep. We'll cover what causes stress responses and what to do about them in more detail in Step 2 of the insomnia programme.

Putting it all together: Adenosine, melatonin and cortisol work together

Both adenosine and melatonin create a drowsy state and send us to sleep. Adenosine simply builds up every moment we are awake and tells us to sleep after we've been awake for a certain number of hours or for too long; it is not influenced by the outside environment. Melatonin, on the other hand, tells us to sleep at a scheduled time of day, and under normal circumstances the timing of its release is influenced by the environmental signals of light and darkness. We can change the timing of melatonin release to suit our needs as we wish by controlling external light and darkness.

The way it's supposed to work is that the combination of about 17 hours' worth of adenosine build-up during the day and the sharp rise in melatonin levels after dark should overcome your awake aroused state and send you to sleep. Ideally by the time the sun has come up and signals to our brain to stop making melatonin we should have slept enough to have eradicated the accumulated adenosine and start over a new day again.

In the morning our internal biological clock should tell our adrenal glands to produce a surge in cortisol and with the sleep-inducing effects of melatonin and adenosine out of the way we should feel refreshed and full of energy.

In the industrialised world both melatonin and adenosine can be in short supply. Electric light in the evening and during the night both inside our homes and coming into our homes from street lighting can delay and reduce melatonin production. Before we had sedentary jobs in offices we would engage in hard physical labour during the day, expending a lot of energy and build up a lot of adenosine to create a strong sleep pressure, so in the past we would be hit by higher levels of sleep-inducing melatonin *and* adenosine soon after dark.

As already mentioned above, ideally you want a rapid surge in melatonin levels to hit you with an intense sensation of sleepiness but this doesn't happen in some people because of their individual biology and excessive artificial light in the evening; add to this a less than optimal level of adenosine due to lack of physical activity and a sedentary lifestyle, then throw in elevated evening cortisol from excessive stress responses and you've lost all the important natural physiological drives to fall asleep. On the insomnia programme in this book you will restore these natural sleep drivers.

In the morning melatonin production may not switch off very quickly due to inadequate bright light; add to this lingering adenosine due to insufficient amounts of sleep and an inadequate rise in energising cortisol due to the adrenal glands being overstressed and taxed and a person is going to be slow to wake up and lack energy in the morning. A morning coffee activates the adrenal glands and temporarily inhibits the effects of adenosine; actually a growing body of evidence suggests that a few coffees a day is positively good for our health but they shouldn't be needed to compensate for inadequate sleep and poor adrenal function.

Insomnia can be a vicious circle

When you don't sleep enough your body fails to completely break down adenosine during the night, making you feel sleepy the following day, so your body will try to compensate for daytime tiredness by asking the adrenal glands to make more cortisol and adrenaline to prop you up; also the tremendous psychological stress and worry insomnia causes will increase the burden on the adrenal glands. Eventually the adrenal glands can become exhausted and unable to produce a strong morning surge of cortisol to give you get up and go, leaving you feeling tired and *even more* stressed about your insomnia. The more stressed you are the harder it is for cortisol to fall to its ideal evening levels, which in turn perpetuates the insomnia by making it hard for you to fall asleep. Instead of cortisol levels rising and falling as they should in people with insomnia and chronic stress cortisol levels tend to 'flatten out' (see Figure 1.2, Unhealthy stress responses and cortisol production).

Subconscious conditioned responses make us sleep

Psychological conditioning plays an important role in activating stress responses; you may have noticed that entering some environments immediately makes you feel upbeat and excited and others immediately make you feel relaxed; perhaps there are places you go where you always sleep well. Have you ever noticed yourself feeling sleepy in your living room but then waking up as you get ready for bed? Our minds make associations based on past experiences and, if your mind associates your bed with good sleep, simply getting ready for bed and lying down will start throwing switches inside your system changing your physiology into sleep mode. If you have insomnia your mind will have developed a negative learned association or conditioned response with your sleeping area and sleeping. You cannot simply 'think' these conditioned responses away; once they are programmed into your protective subconscious stress response system you have to overwrite them with a new conditioned response programme that makes your system shut down and fall asleep as you go to bed. In fact a very good sleeper may actually find it quite difficult to stay awake and lie in bed at the same time, so mental associations also make us sleep and we will use this fact extensively throughout this insomnia curing programme, by doing mental exercises, self-hypnosis exercises, and behavioural techniques.

Declining body temperature makes us sleep

External light sets the timing of the brain's internal biological clock, and our biological clock in turn sends signals to our cells to change the rate of our metabolism or energy production in the evening.

About an hour and a half before falling asleep our metabolism starts to slow down and our internal core temperature falls by about 1°. A change of 1° may not sound like much but this small temperature change causes a significant decrease in the arousal of our physiological system and increases our propensity to fall asleep (see Figure 1.4). In order to fall asleep it is essential that you allow this drop in your internal core temperature to occur, so, for example, a vigorous workout that raises your internal core temperature for perhaps four hours must be avoided too late in the day. Actually you could do a vigorous workout, but only if you are prepared to take a fairly lengthy cold shower or cold bath sufficient to significantly chill your system after your workout.

You must allow your system to cool down for at least 90 minutes before bed; think of your arms and legs as radiators and uncover them to allow your body to dissipate internal core temperature to the outside. In the winter you could switch off your home heating at least a couple of hours before bedtime to help your body to cool down; in hot weather or following exercise in the evening take a long cold shower or cool bath sufficient to give you gooseflesh.

As you can see in Figure 1.4 our internal core temperature continues to decline from an hour and a half before we sleep to its lowest point at about 4 a.m. It's especially important for people who have difficulty staying asleep that they allow their body temperatures to fall and remain low throughout the night. Sleeping with electric blankets switched on and hot water bottles in the bed is not conducive to good sleep, nor is having too many bedclothes. To allow your core temperature to fall during the night you should ideally keep your bedroom quite cool, only minimally use electric blankets and hot water bottles if you have to, just sufficient to offset the initial cold as you get into bed.

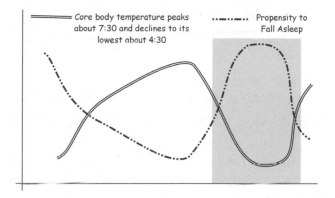

Figure 1.4: The changes in core body temperature throughout the 24 hour sleep–wake cycle

It may not be a particularly practical technique but you can deliberately manipulate your body temperature by heating yourself up with exercise or a warm bath then cooling yourself down with a cold/cool bath or shower at least 90 minutes before you want to sleep.

A gentle way of using temperature changes to influence your sleep is to take a warm (not really hot) bath about two hours before you want to sleep. The bath will warm you up briefly and as long as you allow yourself to cool down afterwards by uncovering your arms, feet and legs and letting your hair dry naturally it can mimic and accentuate the natural drop in body temperature that takes place as part of your 24 hour sleep–wake cycle.

Your brain perceives these deliberately manufactured drops in body temperature as part of your natural sleep system, which can give you a subjective feeling of sleepiness signalling the onset of sleep. If you respond to the feelings of sleepiness by going to bed to sleep it will assist your subconscious to *perceive* the subtle internal signals that tell us when our body is internally winding down and preparing for sleep. Deliberately cooling the body and then going to bed also *programmes subconscious conditioned sleep responses.*

The cooling bath/shower technique can be very useful in hot weather.

The neurotransmitters GABA and serotonin influence sleep and we can safely boost them

Serotonin and GABA are sedating (inhibitory) neurotransmitters that calm and tranquillise the brain; they need to be present in adequate amounts for us to settle our mind and fall asleep.

Serotonin

Not only does serotonin have a sedating effect in its own right but it is also the building block from which the sleep hormone melatonin is made. We can increase the levels of serotonin in our brain by taking the amino acid tryptophan as a supplement. There have only been a few studies into the effect of tryptophan on sleep but they did show promising results, especially in reducing the length of time it takes for a person to fall asleep. Actually the effectiveness of tryptophan as a sleep aid is somewhat hit or miss. It is very helpful to some people and not to others, probably dependent on serotonin status; however even when it is of little help it very rarely causes even mild side-effects.

L-tryptophan → serotonin (serotonin plus darkness) → melatonin → sleep

Studies have shown that the dose of 1 to 2 g of L-tryptophan reduces sleep latency (the time it takes to fall sleep) by approximately half. Tryptophan does not interfere with the normal activity in the brain when you're asleep in the same way that sleeping pills and alcohol do, nor does it lead to dependency when you want to withdraw it. You should definitely consider supplementing tryptophan if you have the combination of insomnia and depression or anxiety.

WARNING: Do not supplement L-tryptophan at the same time you are taking selective serotonin re-uptake inhibitor (SSRI) antidepressants, as it can potentially cause a dangerous condition called serotonin syndrome.

5-HTP versus tryptophan

Tryptophan can be hard to find in the UK and people often substitute 5-hydroxytryptophan (5-HTP), however the latter is not as effective, either as an antidepressant or as a sleep aid.

GABA

Gamma-aminobutyric acid (GABA) is the primary calming, inhibitory neurotransmitter in our brain. It puts the brakes on thoughts, especially worrying, anxious thoughts going around and around in our mind. GABA is also thought to be the primary neurotransmitter involved in sleep processes.

You can increase GABA levels in the brain by supplementing either GABA directly or a compound called L theanine which is extracted from tea.

In my insomnia programme I recommend serotonin and GABA boosting supplements just to assist in initiating better sleeping to overcome insomnia; once you're consistently sleeping well without the aid of sleeping pills you can give them up.

In the next section will look at the biological clock inside our brain that controls our sleep–wake cycles and what we can do to influence it.

How Does Our Biological Clock Affect Sleep Cycles?

Problems with the timing of your sleep cycles

The combination of bright light therapy in the morning, adequate darkness in the evening and specific supplements enables us to influence our melatonin production and our internal 24-hour biological clock which tells our adrenal glands (and numerous other body systems) when to become active and inactive. Not only can we use this as a treatment for insomnia but, as we'll see later when we look at sleep–wake cycles, we can use these things to completely move the timing of your biological clock so that it runs at a time of your choosing that fits your work and social life. Imagine, for example, how useful it would be to turn a teenager from a night owl that doesn't properly wake up till noon into an early bird capable of doing well in a morning mathematics test, or being able stop yourself waking up far too early and having trouble falling asleep too early in the evening, or being able to fit into the schedule of any job you want, etc. For people with bipolar syndrome, where sleep cycle disturbances often play a central role, the potential benefits of these techniques can be enormous.

Moving the timing of your sleep–wake cycle can be reliably done within a week but you will first need to set yourself up with all the necessary blackout blinds, special light bulbs and a bright light device.

As you doubtless already know, we have within us a 24-hour biological clock, also referred to as the circadian (daily) rhythm. This clock regulates many body processes such as our appetite, the time of day we achieve peak mental performance and immune activity, our intestinal movements and our sleep–wake cycles. Here we are only interested in the *sleep–wake cycle* aspect of our circadian rhythm.

You can find nice charts of the times and body systems influenced by our circadian rhythm on Wikipedia if you are interested.

We have an actual biological clock inside our brain which runs our sleep cycles

The biological clock is not just a metaphor, it's a real structure in the brain called the suprachiasmatic nucleus which actually keeps time. This remarkable little structure can keep quite good time; even when it's removed from the body, kept alive and completely isolated from external clues telling it what time of day it is, it will continue to send out its regular scheduled signals. Even without any external signals most people's biological clock keeps quite accurate time and continues on a 24-hour cycle give or take 15 minutes or so.

Throughout the day at specific times the biological clock sends out signals to various parts of the body coordinating the timing of their functions (see Figure 1.5). In the morning the biological clock tells the adrenal glands to produce a surge of cortisol to energise our system; in the evening it tells our metabolism when to slow down, which lowers our core temperature and signals the onset of sleep; it also tells our pineal gland to produce melatonin. The signal to produce melatonin, however, is overridden or stopped as long as light continues to enter the eyes in the evening, and this is one of the things we can control. At the heart of the biological clock is the suprachiasmatic nucleus which sends out signals to the rest of the body to do various things at scheduled times throughout the day. Only the factors affecting sleep that we can control are shown in this simplified figure; the biological clock also tells the bowels to become active about 8:30 a.m. and suppresses bowel function about 10:30 p.m., for example. Bright light exposure sets the timing of the clock.

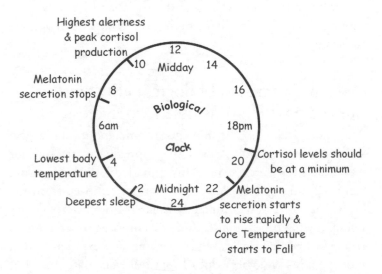

Figure 1.5: The Human Biological Clock

What sets and resets our biological clock

This book is meant to be a self-help book, not a biology lesson, but to understand how to gain control over our internal biological clock, you need to know a little about exactly what external signals reset the timing of the clock.

There are specific cells in our eyes are that do not help us see but whose job is to inform the brain about outside light *levels*; they tell the biological clock when the sun rises and sets. They are called intrinsically photosensitive retinal ganglion cells (sorry, they do not have a simple common name so we will use ipRG cells for short). The existence of the ipRG cells has been known for some time but their function was not understood and their presence was largely ignored until 2002. They are light sensitive but their primary role is not to give us *conscious sight*, they only partially contribute to our visual awareness. On their own they would only give us a very rudimentary form of sight with which we could detect changes in light and dark and a slight sense of movement, but they do not give us fine details or colour. The primary role of the ipRG cells is to inform the biological clock in our brain of the *intensity of outside light* and it is this that resets our biological clock (see Figure 1.6).

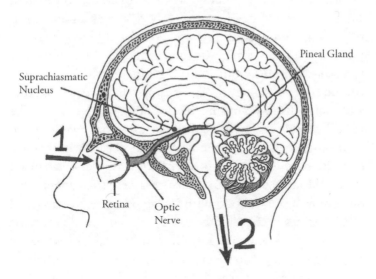

Figure 1.6: The first bright light of the day that enters the eyes sets the timing of suprachiasmatic nucleus (1). This then sends out signals to the body to run our 24 hour cycles (2)

Light entering the eye stimulates the newly discovered light sensitive ganglion cells and tells the biological clock (the suprachiasmatic nucleus) when it's daytime time to 'set' the clock. The biological clock then sends signals at the appropriate times to different systems in the body to tell them when to be active/inactive. This includes the pineal gland that makes melatonin, the adrenal glands that make cortisol in the morning and our core temperature in the evening. Understanding exactly how the ipRG cells and the biological clock work gives us useful techniques to influence our sleep.

The timing of the biological clock is primarily *moved and reset* by exposure to *bright morning light*, that is, the timing of dawn sun. We can use this knowledge and deliberately expose our eyes to a bright light therapy device at a regular time in the morning to set the timing of our sleep–wake cycle to where we want it to be.

The ability of the biological clock to adjust to different sunrise times and day lengths evolved so we can adapt our physiology throughout the year to the different seasons. Natural seasonal changes occur gradually and when we travel great distances quickly our biological clock continues running our physiology (hormones, system, core temperature and metabolism) according to the original time zone. The reset capability of the biological clock is what enables us to adjust to a new time zone and overcome jet lag within a few days; it's hard to imagine but without this reset mechanism we would *never* be able to adjust to a new time zone. Even our stomach can feel odd with jet lag because the activity of our intestines is coordinated on a 24-hour schedule by the biological clock and partially shut down at night while we sleep. Later I will show you techniques to speed up jet lag recovery and even prevent it in the first place (see Part 4).

Another useful finding for our purposes is that the ipRG cells are more prevalent in the lower part of the retina, the part of the eye that receives light from *above*, that is, where the sky is located. This is useful to know because it means that *for maximum efficiency a bright light therapy device should be positioned above your line of sight.*

Perhaps the most interesting finding has been that ipRG cells are most sensitive to blue light, especially blue/cyan light in the range of 460 to 484 nanometres (nm) and that they are hardly stimulated at all by light above 540 nm (see Figure 1.7).

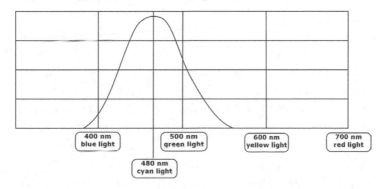

Figure 1.7: Light sensitivity of the ipRG cells

The light sensitivity of the ipRG cells peaks with blue/cyan light then tails off to zero above 550 green light. Red, orange and yellow light doesn't register with these cells. By using only these colours and blocking out all blue/cyan light we create *virtual darkness* in which the biological clock cannot detect any light but we can still see, because the other light sensitive cells in the eye (the ones we see with) still work. Knowing which parts of the light spectrum (colours if you wish) stimulate the ipRG cells is potentially a medical breakthrough and has given rise to some innovative techniques.

First, it gave rise to the development of a more efficient new generation of *blue-light* bright light therapy devices. These devices predominantly emit the blue-light wavelengths that have a bigger effect on the ipRG cells whilst also using less power. The benefit is not just that they are more energy efficient and therefore good for the environment, it also means they can be more pleasant to use. Because they can produce the same or stronger effect on our biology without emitting all the unnecessary wavelengths that have no effect on the ipRG cells they do not have to be as bright (which some people find makes bright light therapy devices unpleasantly dazzling). The new devices can easily be used next to a computer screen, whereas the original devices can make it hard to comfortably view the computer screen.

Second, if it turns out true – as it appears to be – that it is stimulating the ipRG cells that gives bright light its antidepressant effect, then the blue-light devices will have a more efficient antidepressant effect. Bright light therapy has been shown to produce a consistently reliable antidepressant effect on a par with pharmaceutical antidepressants. Hypothetically what may happen is that the absence of (blue) light after dark releases the clamp inhibiting melatonin production and because melatonin is made from serotonin this depletes antidepressant serotonin levels; the application of blue light efficiently stops the conversion of serotonin to melatonin, causing serotonin levels to rise. So hypothetically bright light therapy might be an alternative way of raising antidepressant serotonin, and whatever the mechanism finally turns out to be it does not change the fact that bright light therapy has a proven antidepressant effect and not just for seasonal affective disorder (SAD) winter blues as used to be thought. For a lot more on the antidepressant effects of light see my website www.balancingbrainchemistry.co.uk.

As mentioned above, when sufficient light continues to enter the eyes in the evening it prevents the onset of melatonin production from the pineal gland. In nature this would occur on long summer days; for us, however, it may occur because of excessive bright artificial light in our homes. The useful breakthrough is we now know that it is specifically *only the blue wavelengths of light in the light around us that stimulates the ipRG cells*. Knowing which part of the light spectrum stimulates the ipRG cells and which parts *don't* has led to an incredibly useful technique called *virtual darkness*.

Virtual darkness in the evening

By using special low blue-light emitting light bulbs in the evening and or wearing blue-light blocking (amber) sunglasses we can still see and do things in the evening but as far as our biological clock is concerned we are in total darkness. If you are having trouble imagining virtual darkness, see my sleep website (www.the-sleep-solution.com) for images of the light bulbs and glasses.

In nature sunlight contains all the colours of the rainbow including blue wavelengths, so the ipRG cells know when it's day or night and which season it is by how much blue sky there is and how long the day is. By shielding the eyes from just blue light the ipRG cells are no longer stimulated and the biological clock goes into full night-time mode, initiating the release of melatonin. Remember the ipRG cells' job is to tell the brain when it's day and night, we do not need them to 'see' the world around us, and the other cells in our eyes, the ones that enable us to see, can still function in a low blue-light environment. Virtual darkness essentially tricks the biological clock (the suprachiasmatic nucleus) into believing *all* the light has gone out and darkness has descended.

I would not want to live without my iPad, LED backlit TV, computer monitor and kitchen lights and with virtual darkness we don't have to. Setting up virtual darkness in the evening allows us to carry on our activities as normal, enjoying all the benefits of an artificially lit environment and backlit screens whilst at the same time allowing our body to switch on our melatonin.

At a presentation I gave about my insomnia treatments someone told me that they had hardly slept for three weeks since they bought a large LED backlit TV. These types of TVs give off a lot more blue wavelength light and in her case it appeared to be sufficient to tell her pineal gland that the sun was still shining.

I've seen but not downloaded a free software program that uses the clock inside your computer to know what time of day it was and adjust the brightness and colour scheme of your computer monitor making it brighter and blueish in the morning and dimmer and more yellow in the evening. I hope in the future the potential harm that excess artificial light in the evening is doing will be taken seriously and this type of software would be included in all light-emitting devices in the home.

Removing the blue light from your eyes makes everything appear yellow and feels odd, but only at first, because the brain quickly compensates and you stop noticing anything strange. We'll look at the therapeutic uses of virtual darkness later.

We now have a couple more useful techniques we can use to control our sleep–wake cycles: bright light and virtual darkness.

Total darkness in your sleeping area

Having initiated healthy melatonin production you want to maintain it throughout the night until you are ready to wake up. To achieve this you must completely block out all light entering your bedroom through windows and around the door so that your bedroom is literally pitch black. This is especially important if you are having trouble with waking up too early; some people are supersensitive to early morning dawn light and they need to guard against any light signalling their early rising system it's time to wake up.

Reducing night-time light reduces cancer risk as well

Asking you to make your bedroom totally light tight and changing the lighting in your evening living space to create virtual darkness may sound like a lot of work, so let me tell you the benefits. Cutting out all the light from your bedroom and setting up virtual darkness in your living area will increase your melatonin production and not only will this help you to overcome insomnia and get the best sleep you've ever had but the increased and prolonged melatonin production has numerous other powerful health benefits.

An increasing number of studies link exposure to night-time artificial light and an increased risk in cancer. In 2005 the National Institutes of Health published new research showing that artificial light at night stimulates breast cancer growths in laboratory mice. The study also showed that extended periods of night-time darkness greatly slowed the growth of tumours. Research in the UK (Professor Charalambos Kyriacou at Leicester University) and in Israel (Dr Rachel Ben-Shlomo at the University of Haifa) in 2010 demonstrated that short-term exposure to artificial light increases the risk of cancer; the implication was that turning on the lights during night-time trips to the toilet could increase our cancer risk. The American Medical Association supported further research in 2012 into the possible link between night-time artificial light and increased risk of cancer and obesity. In his book *Great Sleep Reduced Cancer* (2008) Richard Hansler cites over 40 studies demonstrating a link between exposure to artificial light and increased risk in cancer from as far back as 1969 through to 2007.

There is also evidence that the increased production of melatonin experienced by people with total blindness reduces cancer risk by one third (Feychting, Osterlund and Ahlbom 1998). To reproduce this benefit in yourself you would need to spend 12 hours a day encouraging your melatonin production by sleeping eight hours in a totally dark bedroom and spending four hours in the evening in a low blue-light virtual darkness environment. It has been consistently observed that profoundly blind women have proven much less vulnerable to breast cancer (some 30 to 50% less) (Flynn-Evans *et al.* 1991; Hahn 1991). Among profoundly blind men, researchers in Stockholm found a lower incidence of prostate, stomach, colon, rectal, lung and skin cancer (Kukala *et al.* 1999 in Hansler 2008).

Interestingly, blind people who still see light have either had a normal or only a somewhat reduced incidence of these cancers, which is consistent with the theory of melatonin production increasing cancer risk.

There is growing evidence and consensus of opinion that we need to seriously consider that lighting up our evenings in the way we do causes cancers (Feychting *et al.* 1998). It is known, for example, that totally blind people, when no signals of the presence of light reach their brains, have two-thirds the rate of cancer found in sighted people (Feychting *et al.* 1998). It is outside the scope of this book but, briefly, the theory is that melatonin acts as an anti-cancer agent, thus suppressing melatonin levels with artificial night-time lighting increases the incidence of cancer. Assuming this theory is correct you could use the (virtual darkness) techniques discussed in this chapter to increase the amount and the length of time of your melatonin production to be on a par with a blind person and potentially reduce your chances of developing cancer by a third or more.

Increased melatonin production has numerous other health benefits. Melatonin is a powerful antioxidant, protecting the body from ageing free radicals. It has been found to possess 200 per cent more antioxidant power than vitamin E and more powerful than vitamins C and glutathione. Animal studies have shown that melatonin exerts antioxidant protection against heart muscle injury caused by heart attacks. You can find more information and references on the health benefits of melatonin on my website (www.the-sleep-solution.com).

In this book I recommend you use total darkness and virtual darkness both for treating insomnia and for moving badly timed sleep cycles so, rather than repeating the setup instructions, you'll find all the information in Appendix 3, under 'How to Set Up Virtual and Total Darkness'. Please read that section and start to take advantage of these techniques over the next few weeks in readiness for when you start to treat your insomnia or moving your sleep cycle time.

Bright light treatment (BLT)

You probably already have an idea what bright light treatment (BLT) is, but just to make sure, BLT involves keeping a very bright light device in your visual field for 30 minutes or so, usually while you do something like reading, watching television or using a computer. The original bright light devices were called SAD light boxes and consisted of nothing more than powerful fluorescent light bulbs in an large box behind a diffuser. Bright light devices have come a long way since then and are now small compact devices emitting only the specific frequencies that stimulate our ipRG cells. Search online for SAD light box, then click on images and you'll immediately see what BLT is. For instructions on how to perform bright light treatments see Appendix 1.

It turns out that artificial light does the job of entraining our biological clock and signalling to the pineal gland to stop making melatonin just as well as natural daylight sunlight does, which is great because we can reliably create bright artificial light whether we work indoors or whether the sun is shining or not.

Using artificial bright light we can give ourselves a dose of bright light at precisely the best time each day to influence our biological clock and sleep–wake cycles, adjusting them to a schedule of our choosing that best suits our lifestyle.

By combining BLT with the other techniques and protocols described in this chapter you can make waking up and falling asleep too early or too late a thing of the past, you can maximise your sleeping time, wake up more quickly, feeling refreshed, and improve your energy during the day.

Elsewhere in this book only naturally occurring remedies and natural solutions are recommended, however with regards to getting regular therapeutic bright light I suggest that, first – at least in northern climates – man-made bright light devices are superior to natural sunshine hands down! Bright light devices are more reliable and consistent than sunshine. Second, unlike sunlight modern bright light devices do not give off UV (ultraviolet) light which damages the eyes and is linked to an increased risk of cataracts, macular degeneration and other degenerative conditions. Over time the front of the eye becomes yellowed by UV exposure and this yellowing ends up reducing the amount of blue light we receive, contributing to depression and diminishing melatonin production, negatively affecting sleep and cancer risk in the elderly. Even on sunny days I would rather use my bright light device and wear UV protecting sunglasses when I go out. Third, anyone with bipolar/bipolar type II is better off having absolute control over the intensity and duration of their bright light exposure so they can manage the risk of mania/hypomania.

To summarise the multiple potential benefits of bright light therapy:

- It sets the timing of our biological clock, giving us the ability to move our sleep–wake cycles.

- It produces an antidepressant effect, probably increasing serotonin.

- It helps treat insomnia.

- It increases your energy levels and mental performance during the day.

Bright light has been shown to immediately enhance cognitive performance in both students and office workers. Office worker productivity has been shown to improve in brightly lit environments and workspaces illuminated by blue wavelength light have been shown to reduce fatigue and daytime sleepiness (ScienceDaily 2008). The brightness level in a well-lit office or school is unlikely to reach the level at which it could trigger a manic/hypomanic phase in people with bipolar, or disturb the sleep–wake cycle of somebody with delayed sleep phase syndrome (DSPS) who needs to avoid bright light in the evening and so could be adopted in offices and schools without risk. But before doing something *extreme* like attaching blue LED light strips to your employees' computer monitors to wake them up and increase their productivity, one would need to consider the risk of causing mania/hypomania and sleep disturbances in some people.

Bright light therapy is one of those examples of a safe and effective therapy that is completely underutilised because it cannot be effectively patented and made profitable.

Before you move on to the sections on insomnia or sleep cycles there are a couple of supplements that help both conditions that need explaining: very low dose lithium (not the toxic lithium used in pharmaceutical medicine) and very high dose vitamin B-12. These supplements are used in both sections.

Using these two supplements in combination with bright light therapy and virtual darkness is one of the unique aspects of my treatments for insomnia and sleep cycle disorders. They change the effectiveness of the bright light therapy and virtual darkness to give you very powerful tools to control the timing of your biological clock and treat insomnia.

B-12 Methylcobalamin

Earlier I mentioned I use vitamin B-12 in my protocols because of its effects on melatonin production. Let's look at that in a little more detail.

Studies showed that B-12 supplementation directly affects the pineal gland producing a *faster rise in melatonin levels* after dark, and a *faster fall in melatonin levels* in the morning in response to light.

Increasing the rate at which melatonin rises in the blood a couple of hours after dark produces a *stronger feeling of sleepiness*. B-12 also speeds up the rate of decline in melatonin levels in the morning when light starts to enter the eyes helping us to *wake up more quickly*.

On its own supplementing B-12 has little or no effect on sleep; however when combined with bright light and darkness treatment, B-12 significantly accentuates the effects light and dark treatments have on sleep cycles, so you can get a lot more out of them.

What you experience is an increase in the body's connection between your sleep–wake cycle and external light levels. It *intensifies your experience* of melatonin, making you feel sleepier than usual in response to darkness/virtual darkness and more quickly awake in the morning with light.

If you do not normally experience a strong urge to sleep in the evening the combination of B-12 supplementation with bright light in the morning and low/no light in the evening can cause melatonin levels to rise quickly enough to produce an intense wave of sleepiness that hits you like a tsunami. It also helps you wake up in the morning.

A study in Japan (Okawa *et al.* 1997) using just B-12 or a placebo on its own (no bright light exposure) showed no difference between the B-12 group or the placebo group on delayed sleep phase syndrome (DSPS).

Another study, however, published in 1992 (Honma *et al.* 1992) showed that the combination of B-12 and exposure to bright light produced significantly different physiological effects than a placebo and the exposure to bright light. From this and other studies it appears that supplementing B-12 increases the sensitivity of our circadian rhythm to light. Other studies suggest that B-12 probably exerts a direct influence on melatonin production.

A study on a single male student demonstrated the ability of B-12 along with melatonin to reverse and normalise circadian sleep cycles (Tomoda *et al.* 1994).

These experimental observations tally with the anecdotal observation of many people in my practice.

Low dose lithium

Lastly I want to discuss the low dose lithium I use in my sleep treatments both for curing insomnia and moving sleep cycles.

One usually only thinks of lithium as a prescription medication for bipolar syndrome, and in a rather negative light. The high dose of inorganic lithium used by mainstream psychiatry requires frequent monitoring through blood tests because of its toxicity and would be quite inappropriate to use just as a sleep aid. I only treat using naturopathic medicine techniques and do not use toxic medicines, strictly obeying the medical principle of first do no harm.

To supplement the low dose of lithium I use a product called Lithinase, which delivers an organically chelated and absorbable form of lithium. This is an entirely different medicine to the high dose inorganic lithium used in psychiatric medicine. It is safe and side-effect free and can be used by anyone for circadian rhythm sleep disorders and insomnia. Actually, far from being toxic, there is a little evidence that consuming a very low dose of lithium on a daily basis in drinking water may slow the ageing process and extend lifespan.

Lithium has a *direct effect* on one of the principal enzymes involved in the proper regulating of our biological clock and studies have shown that supplementing lithium improves synchronisation of our sleep–wake cycles with the outside world.

Regulating sleep is an important aspect of managing bipolar syndrome and supplementing low dose chelated lithium is doubly beneficial for people with bipolar syndrome as it controls not only sleep cycles but is also an anti-mania mood stabiliser. You'll find more information on this on my website www.balancingbrainchemistry.co.uk.

As a sleep aid I recommend one to three Lithinase with dinner or last thing at night. Dosages above four capsules a day may begin to have sedating effects. (The academic reader can search online for lithium and sleep).

Summary of the things that we can change and influence that control our sleep

- We can influence our melatonin production, when it's produced, how much is produced, for how long it's produced and how quickly its levels rise and fall in the blood.

- We can supplement the amino acid used to make melatonin.

- We can increase adenosine levels through exercise.

- We can move the timing of our biological clock and therefore the entire location of a 24-hour sleep cycle.

- We can change our cortisol production so that it rises in the morning and falls in the evening by changing our stress responses.

- We can influence our core body temperature to help us sleep.

- We can change and rewrite conditioned responses in our subconscious mind that influence our ability to fall asleep (see Part 2).

- We can boost the levels of the sedating neurotransmitters we need to calm the brain and switch off (see Part 2).

PART 2

Overcoming Insomnia

The next section of the book is for people with insomnia. If you bought this book because you want to change the timing of your sleep cycles you can skip this section and go directly to Part 4, Restoring a Healthy Sleep Cycle, now. If you have insomnia the next section is for you, just keep reading.

～ 2.1 ～

What Insomnia is and How to Cure It

Do you have insomnia?

Chronic insomnia is usually defined as taking more than 30 minutes to fall asleep, or being awake for more than 30 minutes during the night, on at least three nights per week for at least six months, and then these sleep patterns causing negative consequences including marked psychological distress, signs of sleep debt (yawning, nodding off, etc.), problems concentrating, learning, remembering things, short-temperedness affecting your social life and work life.

Insomnia is:

- Having trouble falling asleep (called sleep onset insomnia).

- Falling asleep but then having difficulty staying asleep (called sleep maintenance insomnia) where you fall asleep but wake up too often and then have difficulty falling asleep again. (Unfortunately it's possible to have both difficulty with falling asleep and staying asleep.)

- Insomnia can also be having poor *quality* sleep, only having light sleep that does not *satisfy* your sleep needs. The end result of insomnia is lack of restful sleep, the long-term effects of which affect your immune system, your mental performance, emotional well-being and your quality of life.

When you don't get *enough quality sleep* you develop what is called a *sleep debt* and experience tiredness, poor concentration, poor memory, difficulty learning, etc. The tiredness you get with sleep debt from insomnia looks a little different to the tiredness you get from other causes, such as physical exhaustion or an underactive thyroid, for example.

Recognising sleep debt: The tell-tale signs of insomnia

The characteristic signs of sleep debt that distinguish it from tiredness due to other causes and show you have insomnia include:

- frequent yawning

- heavy eyelids

- perhaps closing your eyes momentarily

- nodding off into sleep momentarily, 'head bobbing'

- losing mental focus and contact with what people are saying or what's going on around you and then coming back, because your brain is trying to switch into a mini sleep.

Other signs which may indicate lack of sleep or have other causes include having a short intolerant fuse, weight gain, poor wound healing and other signs of low immunity.

We will see whether you can recover (pay back) sleep debt when we look at what happens when we sleep in Step 3 of the insomnia recovery programme.

The benefits you can expect from this programme and what you'll have to do to achieve them

I wish I could give you some magical herbal insomnia cure that took less than a minute a day to swallow, but there aren't any quick fixes; you must expect to spend five to eight weeks treating your mind and body to fully overcome your insomnia. The first three weeks is largely essential preparation, including pre-loading key sleep-altering nutrients, with the actual treatments beginning in the fourth week. You can expect to see improvements from that point on.

To change your physical body and subconscious mind and overcome insomnia will take about 45 minutes a day for the first couple of months, then 30 minutes per day for the next couple of months to permanently change the way your nervous and hormonal system handles stress responses. Think of it as a dose of medicine that takes 30 plus minutes a day to swallow. The insomnia programme actually creates more than enough extra time for you to do these exercises by making you stay out of bed unless you're actually asleep. All you have to do is follow the programme and your sleep will gradually get better.

I hope you achieve 100 per cent of the goals you're looking for. The programme in this book is very comprehensive, putting together a unique method combining several different approaches aimed at correcting both the physical and subconscious causes that are preventing you from obtaining the sleep you want.

Why sleeping pills are not the answer

- Sleeping pills are only moderately effective and lose their effectiveness with long-term use.

- You can become dependent on sleeping pills.

- Sleeping pills have multiple side-effects, possibly even increasing one's risk of cancer and mortality.

- Sleeping pills may send you to sleep but they actually interfere with the normal activity of the brain and prevent you from being able to achieve deep healthy restful sleep.

- Sleeping pills do not treat the causes of insomnia: they do not produce long-term permanent cures, they do not treat or improve your ability to sleep or change your internal physiology or subconscious psychology. So the insomnia returns when you stop using them.

It's not possible in a book to give you the *individualised* cognitive hypnotherapy techniques that I use in my practice, but the book and accompanying free recordings include general techniques designed to be effective for most people and touch base with many. During private treatment sessions you receive hypnotic techniques to reprogramme the sleep process in your mind based upon your specific and individual sleeping problems, and receive tailor-made exercises matching to the language and way your unique subconscious mind works. For best results I would recommend combining everything in this book with three to five cognitive hypnotherapy sessions, with myself or another therapist who practises cognitive hypnotherapy or NLP and hypnosis.

~ 2.2 ~

Let's Rule Out Medical Causes of Poor Sleep before Treating Insomnia

Before we start the insomnia cure programme we need to rule out treatable physical or mental illnesses that cause insomnia. Once you've done this you can move on to the next section.

Insomnia can have many causes: Why have you got it?
Physical causes of insomnia
If you have long-term insomnia you should have a consultation with your doctor to test for physical causes for your condition. If you are sure you do not have any of these physical causes of insomnia you can skip this section.

Physical causes of insomnia that should be assessed by your doctor and treated by an appropriate healthcare practitioner include:

- angina, asthma, bronchitis, emphysema

- chronic pain, for example, from arthritis

- hypothyroidism, kidney disease, diabetes

- obstructive sleep apnoea.

You must also consider that you may be consuming something stimulating such as caffeine without realising it. Caffeine is sometimes included in painkilling medication, diet pills and steroids. Nasal decongestants, beta blockers and asthma medicines can also have sleep disturbing effects. See Step 2 of the programme.

Below are several conditions that may be helped by alternative medical treatments.

RESPIRATORY ALLERGIES

Respiratory allergies due to dust mites or feathers in one's bedding should be identified and treated. Respiratory allergies to feathers is very common and for this reason I do not recommend feather pillows, duvets, etc. Pillows, in particular, gradually accumulate ever larger populations of dust mites; if you have old feather pillows throw them away and replace them with synthetic filled pillows. Dust mites in the pillow can be killed by frequent washing at 60° or putting the pillow in a freezer for several hours.

OBSTRUCTIVE SLEEP APNOEA

In obstructive sleep apnoea your airways become temporarily blocked, preventing you from being able to breathe. You then wake up to catch your breath and since you're asleep you may not be aware you do this. If you or your partner suspects that you have such a condition you should consult with your doctor without delay as this condition and other breathing problems can significantly increase your risk of developing heart disease.

Conventional medical treatments for this condition include surgically widening your airways, but in over 70 per cent of cases excessive body fat in the throat area contributes to obstructing the airways and so I recommend radical weight loss should be the first line of treatment in anyone with the combination of obstructive sleep apnoea and overweight. Unless you really know what you're doing see a nutritional consultant and your doctor before attempting radical weight loss.

You should also spend at least six months properly learning and practising the Buteyko breathing method; this teaches you to breathe more gently which reduces the likelihood of temporarily collapsing your airways. You can find local Buteyko classes online. I've also seen (but had no clinical experience of) specially made plastic braces that look like night-time teeth grinding shields that you wear at night and are supposed to change the position of your jaw to keep your airways open.

STOMACH ACID REFLUX

Regurgitation from the stomach into the oesophagus can cause sufficient physical discomfort and anxiety to become an organic cause for insomnia. Pharmaceutical treatments for this problem are often of limited benefit, but dietary changes can produce lasting improvements and herbal treatments can also help to manage and eradicate this problem. So consider consulting with a nutritional and herbal consultant such as myself. I have a free page on the dietary recommendations for acid reflux available via e-mail (see www.PeterSmithUK. com for contact details).

RESTLESS LEG SYNDROME

In restless leg syndrome people experience an unpleasant feeling in their legs when they rest causing an irresistible urge to move their legs, often with a jerking motion. Restless leg syndrome can make it difficult for people to fall asleep and it may also disrupt the sleep of anyone else they share a bed with. I've seen complete recovery from this condition from supplementing:

- 50 to 100 mg of B complex

- 200 to 400 mg of magnesium (I typically use magnesium citrate although magnesium malate might produce better results)

- iron (Easy Iron from Higher Nature or Floradix is well absorbed). Studies have observed low levels of iron in the blood and spinal fluid of people suffering from restless leg syndrome and the lower the levels of iron the worse the restless leg symptoms (Allen 2004; Allen and Earley 2007). I'd recommend having a test for serum ferritin levels, a marker for iron stores, if you have restless legs syndrome.

Restless legs syndrome has also been considered to be a sensory disorder and as such it may be treatable using hypnosis and sensory distortion techniques. I have had no clinical experience of treating restless leg syndrome with hypnosis so please contact me if you found it helpful.

Psychological causes of insomnia

After you've addressed physical causes for your insomnia and eliminated sleep disruptors such as stimulating drugs, noise, bright lights, etc., what's left is all in the mind.

Here we are talking about mental health problems such as clinical depression, bipolar syndrome, anxiety disorder, including post-traumatic stress disorder, and phobias such as fear of the dark, for example.

I want to make it clear that the mental causes of insomnia discussed in here are a different category of psychological problems to difficulty falling asleep because of stress, or because you have developed bad sleep habits.

Obviously when mental illness is present you should treat this first or at the same time as addressing insomnia. Sometimes the insomnia corrects itself when you treat the primary mental health problem, sometimes it doesn't, because your subconscious brain has become trained into poor sleep habits and you have now developed insomnia independently on top of the mental health problem, so you need to treat both.

Depression and bipolar syndrome in particular may cause sleep disorders. Delayed sleep phase syndrome with morning tiredness can be common with bipolar syndrome and atypical depression; I suspect this primarily involves imbalances in dopamine. Alternatively waking up abruptly early in the morning can also be a characteristic trait of depression, perhaps involving a deficiency of the calming/ soothing neurotransmitter serotonin. These ideas are purely my own theories and observations; they should not be read as scientific fact and are offered only as useful empirical models upon which to base an initial treatment regime.

DEPRESSION AND INSOMNIA

Insomnia is often associated with depression. Some studies show insomnia precedes depression but this does not mean that insomnia *causes* the depression; perhaps insomnia is an early stage of the depression, just as you have an early incubation stage with a bacterial or viral infection before you experience the full symptoms. The results of studies do not give a clear indication of which is the chicken and which is the egg.

If you do have the combination of depression and insomnia investing in a blue LED bright light device can help both depression and sleep.

BIPOLAR SYNDROME AND INSOMNIA

Bipolar syndrome and sleep disturbances go hand-in-hand and the research suggests that they may share a common origin in the brain. Light therapy can be helpful for the depression side of bipolar syndrome, however it has the potential for inducing mania and so you need to know what you're doing and have already largely stabilised your condition before using this therapy. Interestingly virtual and total darkness techniques have potential therapeutic effects which combat mania and can therefore counterbalance the mania-inducing potential of bright light therapy.

See my website www.balancingbrainchemistry.co.uk for more on treating mental health problems using supplements, bright light and darkness techniques.

Introducing the Insomnia Cure

My treatment programme for successfully overcoming insomnia combines several therapeutic approaches at the same time. Each approach adds something different and together they intensify your natural inbuilt sleep system and remove things that are blocking it.

If you're looking for one single simple and quick thing that you can do, a new pill, some magic herb, one single switch you can change under hypnosis or some such that will deliver a knockout cure to your insomnia I can tell you with some certainty that no such thing exists and you're very likely to be unsuccessful.

On the other hand, if you put the work in and perform all the exercises and techniques prescribed in the insomnia cure that I use in my practice and in this book you really can cure your insomnia within a few weeks. During the time you spend looking for a quick fix you could do this programme and cure your insomnia in the meantime.

Let's begin by considering how good sleepers sleep

The actual moment of falling asleep may only take a few minutes, but even for a good sleeper the *process* of falling asleep is not just throwing a switch, one second you're awake and the next you're asleep. Numerous internal physical and mental processes transition the brain and body from one state to another gradually over more than an hour. Imagine shutting down a movie theatre for the night; you have to switch off heating/cooling systems, ventilation, all electronics in the projection room, food and bar area, the hand dryers in the bathrooms and secure all the exits before the final throwing of all light switches plunges the building into darkness. For a big building this could take quite some time, just like it takes the body time to prepare itself for lights out.

Naturally good sleepers have a set of conscious and unconscious behaviours that move their body and mind into the right place for them to fall asleep without even thinking about it. They also have healthy attitudes and emotions about sleep that don't create any problems for them to fall asleep, they may not even know that they have internal attitudes and beliefs about sleep: it is just something they do without even thinking about it. Their mind, nervous system and stress hormones are all naturally in sync with the time of day and begin to wind down prior to bedtime. The intention of the insomnia treatment in this book is to turn you into one of those people, a good natural sleeper.

As the day winds to a close the nervous system in a good sleeper swings away from the alert, stressed, switched on active state progressively toward a relaxed condition; it is unhindered by any worry or anxiety about being able to fall asleep. Levels of the stress hormones adrenaline and cortisol decline, their blood pressure and core body temperature begin to go down. Their conscious wakeful alertness begins to wane and levels of the sleep hormone melatonin begin to rise. Their subconscious mind picks up on these clues automatically and without them even having to think about it their subconscious drives appropriate behaviours, it picks them up off the sofa, gets them into the bathroom to brush their teeth and before they know it they are in bed with their head on the pillow. Then they can simply effortlessly fall asleep without even thinking about it; even if they wake up during the night, which is quite common at the end of a dream cycle, or to go to the bathroom, they effortlessly fall asleep again straight away.

You could describe all the things that good sleepers do naturally as a kind of winding down, sleep preparation ritual, and the good news is that you can train or retrain your mind how to do all of this automatically again. As I will discuss later we can train ourselves to do things automatically simply by repeatedly practising the thing we want to happen; this gives us one of the first practical techniques we will use to instil in you the same well-functioning sleep processes that automatically make good sleepers sleep. You will add hypnotic exercises to this that train your mind to recognise and eventually automatically respond to the subtle clues your body gives our mind that it is time to initiate the winding down sleep behaviour rituals. You will also do hypnotic exercises to intensify the innate feelings of being sleepy, and other exercises to make your mind see yourself falling asleep rather than what it may currently do (which is see you lying in bed not asleep with insomnia).

With other hypnotic exercises you will transform and switch off unhelpful psychology buried in your subconscious that can keep you awake. For example, you may be so anxious about not being able to sleep and feeling awful the next day that you are too stressed to fall asleep. There are many psychological obstacles like this that can maintain the insomnia. The good news is that although these unhelpful psychological processes can have very powerful effects they are not in themselves special or powerful thought processes and there are effective techniques from cognitive hypnotherapy and NLP that can reprogramme the mind to remove these problem ways of thinking.

Components of the insomnia cure

1. Practising and rehearsing good sleep behaviours to relearn how to sleep

In this programme I take as a starting point the CBT sleep programme that has been properly researched and developed over a couple of decades at Harvard and Massachusetts Medical Schools and helped tens of thousands of people to overcome insomnia, producing results in 90 per cent of patients (Galuszko-Wegielnik *et al.* 2012; Jacobs *et al.* 2004). This part of the treatment works by making changes to your sleeping behaviour, the mental associations you have with sleep and undergoing a training programme to teach the nervous system to relax deeply and efficiently. Some of you may not believe that simple behavioural changes could cure *your* insomnia but it has been scientifically proven that we all can reprogramme the associations our subconscious brain makes by performing behavioural exercises/therapy. In one study it was shown that six hours of behavioural training improved sleep quality and speed of onset. Interestingly, the ten-month follow-up of this study showed that better long-term results were obtained from the behavioural training when sleeping pills were disallowed during the training (see Hauri 1997; Morin *et al.* 2006). The CBT sleep programme contributes an invaluable way of establishing a bedtime schedule that changes your subconscious brain's connection to your bed from a place where you have insomnia and don't sleep to a place that you associate with sleeping.

By changing our behaviour we can change our subconscious mental programming. You may not want to believe that simply changing your behaviour and rehearsing rituals over and over again can influence the way you think; your conscious mind may think, as mine does, that you have independent free will and make up your own mind in decisions about things. We now know from extensive psychological studies that simply by deliberately changing our behaviour we can challenge and change our mental attitudes and that when we repeat the same action over and over again our subconscious mind learns how to do this action and then performs it for us automatically in the background without us even having to consciously think about it any more. The conscious brain can only focus on and coordinate a few things at one time; what enables us to do a multitasking complex activity is our subconscious brain. When we repeatedly consciously practise something our subconscious brain gradually learns how to do the new complex activity and can then perform it in the background, freeing up your conscious mind to think about other things. When a child first learns how to walk, it struggles to coordinate the sensations of keeping the body upright and position/movements of its arms and legs. Eventually we become so good at doing all of this that we can run without even thinking about it and have our conscious minds freed up to make life or death decisions about which way to run. Other classic examples of this process are driving a car, riding a bicycle, swimming, knitting, etc. When you first learn to do these things you had to concentrate consciously on each step, you may have been unable to manage to do everything together at the same time and had to begin with taking baby steps, only one thing at a time. Now, however, you can drive a car and do many other complicated things without even thinking about it.

Our subconscious minds take over running repetitive day-to-day behaviours with amazing efficiency and over the next few weeks you going to train your unconscious mind to take over sending you off to sleep with the same amazing efficiency it does all the other things.

An interesting and very important aspect of the subconscious brain is that once it has learned a new skill it tends to never forget it. So once you have learned to drive, swim or ride a bicycle you've installed that programme for life. If you learned how to do something properly in the beginning it will carry on working in the usual way; but if when you learned how to do something you learned bad habits you will carry on repeating these bad habits again and again; the classic example of this is picking up a bad habit when you're learning to drive that stays with you indefinitely.

Left alone, subconscious programmes will carry on working more or less unchanged; they are not, however, set in stone and we can add new information to what we have previously learned or even overwrite learned programmes if we put in enough effort. In this way we can improve and develop our existing skills; however, we can also pick up and learn new ways of doing things that that are *undesirable* and corrupt the original well-functioning programming. These undesirable modifications will continue running unchanged until they are overwritten and this is what you will do during this treatment. The subconscious brain plays a central role in running the processes of falling asleep automatically for us in the background. If you're reading this book you doubtless have a sleep problem and carry some stress and anxiety about it. Our brains have been built to be acutely sensitive to anything that feels stressful or threatening, and in order to keep us safe we have highly involved systems in our subconscious brain to learn where the stress or potential threats lie. This system is designed to keep you safe in the jungle but it can cause problems blocking our ability to sleep. Your subconscious mind will have learned that your bedroom and bed are stressful places and will actively try and *prevent* you from falling asleep because falling asleep in a stressful place could be dangerous. The problem is that some of the simple parts of our brains are unable to distinguish between some of our modern mental stresses and worries and real life or death danger. The good news is that we can re-educate these parts of a brain and reinstall healthy programmes.

Chronic or long-term insomnia often develops from a period of short-term poor sleeping due to stress, trauma, illness, work or social demands. You may have been a good sleeper in the past, with healthy sleep behaviours being run for you automatically in the background by your subconscious mind without you even having to think about it. Then, because of circumstances, you may have gone through a period of poor sleeping; during this time your subconscious sleep programmes can become reprogrammed in a way that stops you sleeping properly. Your subconscious now associates lying in bed with *not* sleeping and as bedtime looms it provokes thoughts and feelings of worry and anxiety that stimulate stress (fight or flight) responses, releasing adrenaline and cortisol, the exact opposite to what it should be doing. Once insomnia has developed it is common to develop additional problems from stressing about the problem and worrying whether you will ever sleep properly again. Any health problem can cause stress, but with insomnia stressing about not being able to sleep compounds the problem and can make it significantly harder to fall asleep.

All the above problems can be changed, reprogrammed and overcome using the behavioural, hypnotic and NLP techniques in this book. As you will see, during my insomnia treatment in addition to psychological treatments you will also incorporate several physical treatments, correct physical problems and intensify the pressure to sleep and get you back into good sleeping.

2. Directly installing natural sleep programmes and uninstalling faulty beliefs that are preventing good sleep

Effective as the behavioural techniques above are at retraining your mind to become a good natural sleeper, when it comes to working with errors programmed into the subconscious mind CBT behavioural techniques have now been superseded by cognitive hypnotherapy and NLP techniques which give us more direct tools to cure insomnia.

The subconscious mind is often remote and inaccessible to our conscious thinking brain; the most direct technique developed to *access and interact* with the subconscious mind is hypnosis and when combined with NLP it is possible to make lasting therapeutic changes. In my practice I use a technique called cognitive hypnotherapy, which has as one of its hallmarks that there are no predetermined hypnotic scripts, no 'one size fits all' hypnotic suggestions for curing insomnia. The way one person describes how they experience, see or feel their sleep problem and how they see good sleep is unique and quite different to another person's. To create efficient lasting change, cognitive hypnotherapy uses the specific language, thinking structures and patterns used by a person's individual mind. The individual mental qualities and language structures a person uses to think are incorporated (we call this *wordweaving*) into the treatment to ensure the hypnotic interventions 'speak' to your unique subconscious. The free recordings that accompany this book unfortunately cannot be tailor-made to your unique subconscious mind. To compensate for this the recordings incorporate multiple permutations, essentially saying the same thing several times in different ways, relying on the inbuilt ability of your subconscious to find a suitable match with one of the permutations and make use of it. (See Contact Details and Getting the Free Recordings.) This isn't as crude or difficult as you might imagine; remember that within your body and mind are natural self-healing systems developed over hundreds of thousands of years of evolution *that are trying to help you* get well again. You already possess within you natural sleep processes that are trying to work properly. Even if there are parts of your subconscious mind behaving in a way that makes it hard for you to sleep properly there are other large parts of you that want you to sleep and want this programme to work; those parts will pick up the bits from the recordings that resonate with your mind and make them work for you. In addition to the recordings there are mental exercises in each step.

3. Intensively train how to switch on relaxation responses in your nervous system

Some versions of the CBT sleep programme I've seen published grossly underutilise the potential of the relaxation response to treat insomnia, with basic instructions and dedicating only a short amount of time to mastering this technique. When we over-produce stress responses we over-produce the stress hormone cortisol at the wrong time of day. Cortisol is a stimulating hormone supposed to give us a surge of energy and peak performance in the morning; when we produce too much cortisol late in the day it maintains an active aroused metabolism and makes it hard for our bodies to fall asleep. We need to prevent the overproduction of cortisol in the evening. Training the relaxation response very efficiently removes this problem when it's done properly and can re-establish the healthy morning surge and night-time decline of cortisol that helps to create a normal sleep–wake cycle. The use of bright light therapy in the morning enhances the psychical rise and fall of cortisol and improves your ability to wake up in the morning and fall asleep in the night.

The problem with training the relaxation response has always been the enormous amount of time one has to put into the training before it makes *permanent curative changes*. I have been using the health benefits of the relaxation response for over two decades in my practice and over the years I've tried various ways of cutting corners to reduce the amount of time it takes to obtain the full therapeutic effects. Unfortunately every shortcut I tried diminished the results and I am now adamant that there is *no substitute* to putting in many hours of practice over many days. In my insomnia cure you have to do half an hour a day of deep relaxation for 100 consecutive days, that's a full 50 hours of training, much more than typically advocated in the basic CBT programme. This intensive and long training programme has absolutely consistently delivered *radical and permanent therapeutic changes* in my clients' nervous systems.

4. Reducing blue evening light to maximise and bring on melatonin production

Another powerful resource you will use to enhance your sleep system is to control the specific frequencies of light that influence the production of melatonin, your natural inbuilt sleep inducing hormone. Increasing your night-time production of melatonin helps you to fall asleep and stay deeply asleep throughout the night. With the light control techniques in this book you will learn how to maximise your melatonin production and coax every last drop out of your pineal gland.

5. Boosting your brain's calming neurotransmitters to help you sleep

My background in working with balancing brain chemistry for depression, bipolar syndrome, anxiety and addictions has introduced to my sleep cure the use of diet and supplements to boost levels of the brain-calming neurotransmitters GABA and serotonin. Serotonin not only calms and soothes the mind, it is also the building block of melatonin, our brain's sleep-promoting hormone. One of the important roles GABA plays in our brains is to put the brakes on and stop persistent worrying thoughts going around and around in the mind; after an appropriate amount of time a worrying thought should be stopped and GABA literally puts the thoughts to bed. Both GABA and serotonin levels can be safely boosted in the brain using natural remedies, at least initially, to help kick-start deep healthy sleep. These remedies do not carry the same risk of dependency and side-effects that sleeping pills possess. When insomnia is directly due to depression and or anxiety, boosting these neurotransmitters may be central to your recovery.

6. *Physical activity to increase adenosine in the blood*

Last, but by no means least, you can increase the amount of physical activity and exercise you do during the treatment programme. This builds up a more powerful pressure to sleep at the end of the day.

Putting it all together

In my insomnia programme I use a tried and tested *cognitive behavioural* programme that has been developed over the past 20 years and helped thousands of people as the backbone and integrate this with *cognitive hypnotherapy and NLP* techniques that reprogram your mind on a deeper subconscious level. Training the *parasympathetic relaxation response* of the nervous system is included. It is often underutilised in other insomnia treatments but in my programme is developed (to the point of overkill some might say). I defend my stance on how much relaxation training is required because the level of training my treatments demand consistently delivers results. In the case of insomnia it will remove the problem of evening cortisol from the table.

The cognitive behavioural techniques change how you think (the cognitive part) about sleep and your sleep behaviour; you will learn how to pay attention to your body's natural sleep and then respond to it with the right behaviour. These techniques primarily target the conscious mind and the belief is that as you see your sleep improving your subconscious mind will start to reprogram its understanding. This does work, however, it can become stuck and undone by strong and entrenched programming buried in the subconscious. In the hypnotic/self-hypnotic state one can interact with the subconscious mind and reprogram unhelpful thinking. With cognitive hypnotherapy techniques it's possible:

- to rewrite negative programmes in the subconscious. It turns out that our memories and perceptions are plastic and can be remodelled by bringing them up to the surface, a bit like opening a stored file, changing something and then putting the file back. The rest of the mind accepts the alteration and changes the way you behave and see things. It's also a bit like uninstalling and then reinstalling a computer program that is not working the way you want it to. You can actually do this to yourself with the recordings for this programme or, better still, get a tailor-made treatment based upon your individual story by having three or four sessions with a cognitive hypnotherapist.

- to install positive ways of thinking that counteract the negative programmes. I sometimes think of this as installing an antivirus program that works its way through your system neutralising bad software programs.

- that as your cognitive mind increases its awareness of your natural sleep systems you will be able to programme this awareness and the appropriate behaviour into your subconscious mind, which will then take over management of your sleep so that it works effortlessly and automatically in the future. All you have to do to get there is to install the new programming by following the exercises.

It has been shown that to be successful you do not have to be in a deep state of trance to benefit from hypnotic suggestions, and you should easily be able to achieve a state of hypnotic trance perfectly adequate to make this technique work for you.

Every single technique in this insomnia programme is important; do it all and you will get results. Not only do each of the different techniques have a different function and address a different part of you but they also reinforce each other and added together they create a much more powerful and effective cure.

Putting it all together you will:

- increase melatonin levels naturally with virtual and total darkness techniques

- increase sleep-inducing neurotransmitters serotonin and GABA with nutritional supplements

- eradicate the problem of excess evening cortisol keeping you awake by intensively training the parasympathetic relaxation response

- combine the best of cognitive behavioural therapy, cognitive hypnotherapy and NLP techniques to enable you to reprogramme and reinstall their working programmes into your subconscious, enabling you to switch off the wake system in your brain and switch on the sleep system automatically.

By combining all these techniques you should have everything you need to make your insomnia history.

Outline of the insomnia programme steps
Step 1
This step is largely about making preparations.

- Stock your sleep medicine chest.

- Start making your bedroom light tight.

- Keep a record of how you've slept for seven days.

- Practise the daily breathing meditation technique.

- Start the self-hypnosis programme, telling your subconscious to see yourself sleeping well in the future.

Step 2

This step is all about eliminating the stress responses and elevated cortisol that are keeping your system awake.

- Learn about and eliminate all the things which can interfere with good sleeping.

- Learn about and understand how to control your stress responses.

- Perform mental exercises to help you let go of anger or the stresses of the day and fall asleep.

Step 3

- Learn about sleep and health.

- Start some of the supplements to pre-load with them before starting the next phase.

- Perform mental exercises to let go of stress by clarifying your goals and programming your subconscious mind to figure out solutions to your problems while you dream.

- In Recording 3 are exercises where you practise seeing yourself going through the steps as you transition to bed and remain sleepy throughout the process.

Step 4

In this step the insomnia treatments begin in earnest.

- Start all the bedroom scheduling techniques to retrain your subconscious brain.

- Start performing bright light therapy in the mornings and rigidly imposing virtual darkness in the evenings, and total darkness in your bedroom.

- Add supplements which induce better sleep.

- Perform a mental exercise to practise feeling sleepy.

- The Step 4 recording includes a mental exercise to diminish and eradicate feelings and beliefs that you are stuck with insomnia and see its grip on you breaking up and letting go.

Step 5

- Learn how to evolve the bedroom scheduling techniques; increase the amount of time you sleep each night and build on your progress.

- Learn about sleeping pills and their outcome.

- Learn advanced relaxation techniques.

Step 6

- Continue increasing the number of hours you sleep.

- Continue weaning yourself off sleeping pills.

- Repeat and consolidate any of the exercises or recordings you found useful from the previous steps.

- Continue doing a daily parasympathetic relaxation response training to complete 100 days.

- Recording 6 includes instructions to project the improvements and successes you've achieved so far continuing into the future for the rest of your life.

- Sleep well for the rest of your life!

PART 3

The Insomnia Cure Step-by-Step Treatment Programme

Table 3.1 Outline of the Insomnia Programme Steps

Step 1 (1–2 weeks)	Stock up on the sleep remedies and equipment you'll need to move your sleep cycles and cure your insomnia.	Make a start on making your bedroom completely light tight to maximise your melatonin production and prevent your biological clock waking you up when dawn light hits your bedroom windows.	Make a seven-day record (the sleep diary) of how you've slept to measure your progress against in the future.	1. Practise a daily breathing exercise to train your nervous system to relax. 2. Start hypnotically programming your subconscious to see yourself overcoming your insomnia and sleeping well in the near future.
Step 2 (1–2 weeks)	Learn about what provokes the stress responses that over-produce the stress hormone cortisol in the evening and prevent you from falling asleep.	Start practising the daily parasympathetic relaxation response to permanently train your nervous system how to switch off stress responses.	Learn about anything and everything from diet to temperature that interferes with sleep and start eliminating them.	Learn and perform mental exercises to help you let go of anger or the stresses of the day which may prevent you from being able to fall asleep.

Step 3 (1 week)	Start taking some of the key sleep-enhancing supplements to pre-load them into your system before starting Step 4.	Learn about sleep and health.	Perform mental exercises to: 1. Diminish stress by clarifying the nature of your problems and goals and the immediate steps you need to take to make things better. 2. Programme your subconscious mind to work out solutions to your problems while you sleep.	Hypnotically programme your subconscious to go through the steps of going to bed and falling asleep without provoking a stress response because of anxiety about sleeping which releases more stress hormones.
Step 4 (1–2 weeks)	In this step the insomnia treatments begin in earnest, and you start all the behavioural bedroom scheduling techniques to retrain your subconscious associations with sleep. Add several new supplements to increase levels of neurotransmitters that induce better sleep.	Start performing bright light therapy in the mornings to 'stimulate' your biological clock and rigidly impose virtual darkness before you sleep and total darkness in your bedroom to increase melatonin production.	Perform mental exercises to practise *inducing* the feeling of being sleepy.	Hypnotically programme your unconscious mind to eradicate negative beliefs that you are stuck with insomnia and cannot overcome its grip on you.

Step 5 (Complete 100 days of relaxation. This gives you time to permanently adjust your sleep physiology to longer and better sleeping, and wean yourself off sleeping pills.)	Increase and progress the amount of time you sleep each night at the right pace to allow your sleep physiology to adjust gradually.	Learn about sleeping pills and how to come off them.	Learn advanced relaxation techniques to release emotional tension.	
Step 6	Continue increasing the number of hours you sleep and conditioning your physiology to maintain good quality sleeping habits. Continue weaning yourself off sleeping pills.	Continue doing a daily parasympathetic relaxation response training to complete 100 days and permanently train your nervous system to drop stress responses at will.	Repeat and consolidate exercises and recordings you found useful or challenging from the previous steps.	Hypnotically programme your unconscious mind to project the progress you've made continuing into the future and becoming a good sleeper for the rest of your life.

∼ Step 1 ∼

Increasing Your Natural Melatonin and Gathering the Supplies You'll Need

You can start two parts of the sleep recovery programme straight away:

- First, start today recording a sleep journal over the next seven days. The sleep journal needs to be completed before you can proceed with Step 4 so you need to complete it within the next three weeks; it only takes a couple of minutes a day.

- Start training your parasympathetic (relaxation) response as soon as possible. The parasympathetic response training starts to produce initial benefits within weeks but the effects build up over three months, so the sooner you start the sooner you reap the full benefits. If you want to get started today you can find comprehensive written instructions in the self-help pages of my website www.PeterSmithUK. com or wait for the free MP3 recording I will send you via e-mail; simply request Better Sleep recording 1 via e-mail (see Contact Details and Getting the Free Recordings). The recordings not only guide you through how to switch on your parasympathetic relaxation response, each recording also guides your mind through mental exercises to engage your subconscious to help you sleep.

Your goals in Step 1

(Give yourself 1–2 weeks to complete this phase.)

1. Purchase the sleep-promoting remedies. See 'Shopping list for the insomnia cure' on page 91.

2. Start training your nervous system how to switch on the relaxation response every day. On the free recordings you are guided through the process of putting your body into a deeply relaxed condition.

    Following the recordings you will induce a relaxation response which takes care of this important part of the insomnia cure then, once you're in a deeply relaxed state, you will be guided through a mental exercise to make changes in your subconscious. In each step of the treatment you will do a different mental exercise with a specific function to overcome insomnia and make you a good sleeper.

3. As well as listening to the recording and switching on a relaxation response on each step you will do an exercise to address specific problems that can prevent healthy sleeping. The first daily exercise of the programme is performing a breathing meditation exercise; you'll find instructions for two breathing exercises and how to choose the right one below.

4. Start setting up a totally dark light-tight bedroom and make a start on reducing your exposure to artificial (blue wavelength) light in the evening. This will increase the production of your sleep hormone melatonin and maintain it throughout the night.

5. Start increasing your physical activity/exercise, even just walking an extra ten minutes a day can start to make a difference.

6. In this first step you will also learn about the sleep remedies.

Every part of this programme performs an important and specific function, so *do the whole programme, don't just pick out the parts you think apply to you*. Even if one of the techniques does not deal with the main cause of your problem they all contribute some sleep-inducing effect and reinforce each other.

Making a sleep diary

The sleep diary is just a simple, subjective estimating of your current sleep situation that you will use later to determine the correct time for you to go to bed and get out of bed. It only takes a minute in the morning to complete your diary, within one hour of rising, and simply guess the times to the nearest 5–10 minutes. If you miss a day it's okay – just do it tomorrow.

If you have insomnia you'll probably already be thinking about how much sleep you are getting and clock watching; paradoxically doing this makes it even harder to fall sleep. During the first week of the insomnia cure programme you need to keep a sleep diary (Table 3.2) in order to carry out the sleep scheduling techniques you'll use in the rest of the programme. Sometimes keeping a sleep diary helps people to see that they're actually sleeping more than they thought; more often than not, however, it makes the clock watching problem temporarily worse. All you can do is try not to get more stressed by keeping a sleep diary and accept it's just a short-term step you need to take to move you forward. You don't have to worry about being very accurate as it only has to be a subjective guide; just do the best you can and within a few weeks on the rest of the programme your sleep diary should become irrelevant anyway.

Table 3.2 Sleep diary

	Day 1	Day 2	Day 3	Day 4	Day 5	Day 6	Day 7
What time did you go to bed?							
What time did you turn the lights out?							
About how long did it take you to fall asleep? (½, 1, 1½ hours, etc.)							
About how long were you awake during the night altogether? (½, 1, 1½ hours, etc.)							
What time did you wake up in the morning?							
Add up how many hours you slept last night							

When you've completed the entries for the week, use a calculator to add up all the hours you slept over the last week and divide that total number by seven to work out how many hours you sleep on average per night; we'll use this number in Step 4.

The insomnia remedy medicine chest

In this insomnia programme, to enhance the power of the behavioural therapy, the hypnotherapy, the bright light and darkness techniques, you will combine the sleep-inducing remedies below to kick-start good sleeping.

L-tryptophan

Tryptophan is converted in the brain into serotonin, which has a natural antidepressant effect; serotonin is in turn converted into melatonin, our primary sleep-inducing hormone.

There is evidence that a dose of 1000 mg of L-tryptophan reduces the time it takes to fall asleep. I've seen studies that suggest there is no evidence that tryptophan helps you to stay asleep, however other studies show blood levels of tryptophan are low in people with primary insomnia and that tryptophan significantly increases the depth of the deep sleep phase we have in the beginning of the night. My personal experience is that tryptophan gives you a deeper and more refreshing sleep.

Studies suggest that even when tryptophan is prevented from being converted into serotonin (and therefore melatonin) it still improves sleep (Wyatt *et al.* 1970), which I find interesting because I have often found it beneficial to combine tryptophan and melatonin supplements.

Just in case you're wondering, it is perfectly safe to take both tryptophan and melatonin together at the same time; the combination doesn't produce some kind of dangerous excess melatonin syndrome. Before I understood how to use B-12, low dose lithium, along with bright light and darkness therapy, I would regularly combine tryptophan, melatonin and zinc to fight my sleep phase disorder; there are no contra-interactions between these remedies discussed in the literature.

Dosage: 1000–2000 mg one hour before you go to bed at least 2½–3 hours after eating any protein. You may get results with 500 mg but I doubt you reach a therapeutic threshold.

Caution: Do not take tryptophan at the same time as anti-depressants; see my website www.balancingbrainchemistry. co.uk for more details.

B-12
As already discussed B-12 speeds up the rate at which melatonin is produced at night, which precipitates a more intense desire to fall asleep.

B-12 is not only completely safe to take at high doses but it is in fact very good for you because it reduces homocysteine, a harmful chemical that causes damaging inflammation throughout our body (Clarke *et al.* 1998; Huang *et al.* 2012; Yakut *et al.* 2010).

Dosage: 1000–5000 mcg held under the tongue for several minutes. You must choose the right form of B-12 (methylcobalamin not cyanocobalamin) and also the right type of sublingual preparation to bypass the intestines. If you don't get these two things right you will not get the benefits. See the Appendix 2 for more information.

Lithium
As already discussed lithium improves the healthy functioning of our biological clock to establish healthy sleep cycles; when functioning well and combined with adequate bright light

during the day and darkness during the night your biological clock will change your internal physiology so that you are fully awake during the day and fully asleep during the night.

Dosage: Lithinase from Progressive Laboratories (available from iherb.com): 1 capsule with breakfast, 1–2 capsules with dinner.

Zinc

Zinc is an excellent and safe sleep aid; it can also have a calming and antidepressant effect. It can be difficult to absorb from the intestines so always buy good quality zinc chelated supplements. Amino acid chelates were the best but have now been superseded by the Food State technology sold in the UK by Nature's Own or Cytoplan, and the True Food technology sold by Higher Nature. Unfortunately I am not familiar with the brands of Food State supplements in other countries. Look for brands with the name Food State in their information and you will see they are blended with *S. cerevisiae* in the ingredients. In the USA I recommend Mega Food (available from iherb.com).

These supplements have been processed through live (safe) yeasts so that they end up as a true concentrate of how the mineral actually occurs in nature in real foods. Another great advantage these types of supplement give us is that you can take Food State zinc on an empty stomach last thing at night without problems; if you take a non-Food State regular zinc supplement on an empty stomach it can make you feel nauseous. Single doses over 60 mg in almost any format can induce nausea.

Dosage: To help your sleep try a dose of 40–50 mg last thing at night if you're using a regular zinc amino acid chelate or half that dose if you can get Food State supplements. To metabolise zinc you need B-6 but the problem with taking much B-6 late at night is that it can induce such vivid dreams that it will disturb your sleep. The solution is to take a small dose of B-6, about 5–10 mg combined with your zinc works well. I recommend half a Nature's Own Food State B-6 tablet or a Food State B complex. If you can't get the Food State supplements, taking a regular B complex with dinner should provide sufficient B-6.

On the issue of safety, regular zinc supplementation can suppress your iron and copper levels; this is easily prevented by supplementing a low dose of iron and copper. For this reason most manufacturers add iron or at least copper to their zinc supplements. Supplementing 80 mg in total every day can cause health problems but only after several years. A single dose of more than 550 mg can be poisonous but you would probably vomit most of it up fairly quickly.

Zinc in general boosts the immune system, especially with regard to fighting viruses; however, high doses of zinc supplements, above say 30 mg, may actually diminish your immune system when fighting a heavy bacterial infection such as a chest infection. See my Natural Antibiotics and Immune Boost Doc, which are available free from my self-help pages on my websites (see Contact Details and Getting the Free Recordings).

Magnesium

Numerous studies have demonstrated magnesium to possess a hypnotic or sleep-benefiting effect. Compared to the above remedies this effect is mild yet still valuable. Several studies have also shown that that the diet in western developed countries is often magnesium deficient.

Take 400–600 mg with dinner as a sleep (and general health) aid.

Magnesium oxide is cheap but very poorly absorbed; don't use it. Magnesium citrate is a good value, well-absorbed, general purpose version. Magnesium malate would be the version to choose if you suffer from neurological or muscular pain such as fibromyalgia.

GABA

GABA is an inhibitory neurotransmitter; it puts the brakes on anxious, worrying thoughts going around and around in the mind and has a general calming effect. If anxiety, racing thoughts or stress are causing insomnia try GABA, or theanine which boosts GABA levels, as sleep aids.

Dosage: The therapeutic dose of GABA for insomnia may need to be fairly high, from 1000 to 3000 mg.

Theanine 100–200 mg taken shortly before retiring.

Omega-3 oils

Higher doses of omega-3 oils can make one feel very sleepy and can be used as an occasional sleep aid. The sleep-inducing effect comes on within several hours after dosing. Since omega-3 oils also have mood-stabilising (anti-mania) effects they are a potentially useful option to help quickly shut your system down during a manic episode.

There can be a downside to doing this, however; if you suffer from depression or bipolar syndrome, exceeding the dose which you have established *helps* your mental health problem may slightly intensify or *induce* a mild depression the following day. This negative effect is temporary however, only lasting a few days at most, and may be worth putting up with for the sleep benefits.

You could try the heavy-handed dose of fish oils at a time when your depression is in remission so you gain an understanding of the effects of this sleep-inducing technique.

Research has shown that omega-3 oils have a similar mood-stabilising mechanism of action as lithium on bipolar, albeit not as powerful. However omega-3 oils do not regulate our 24-hour biological clock the same way lithium does. So fish oil may benefit insomnia (sleep quality and quantity) but not sleep rhythm disorders. With bipolar syndrome always pre-load omega-3 oils into your brain for a week or so *before* starting bright light treatment to minimise the small but potentially serious risk of mania.

Exercise

Being physically active increases the body's production of *adenosine*, which increases sleep pressure, helping you to fall asleep at the end of the day. Have you ever noticed that you slept like a log on days when you were very physically active (long hikes, moving house and carrying lots of boxes, etc.) This is because a by-product of the body metabolising energy is to produce adenosine and the more energy you expend the more adenosine you build up. It may not be at all practical but if there's any way that you can do a genuinely large amount of physical activity in the early stages of Step 4, when we begin to apply several other sleep-inducing techniques it will add even more pressure to get you started sleeping better.

Even more moderate amounts of exercise, say 20 minutes vigorous walking, have been shown to significantly improve the sleep of people with chronic insomnia, shortening the length of time it took to fall asleep and increasing the length of time people stayed asleep (Passos *et al.* 2010).

You probably just have to fit in exercise whenever you can, however if you have the choice try a strenuous workout session of at least 20 minutes, or sufficient to make you feel hot, about three hours before you want to sleep. As your body temperature cools down it acts as an additional signal telling the body to sleep (Horne and Staff 1983). Raising your core temperature through exercise immediately before trying to sleep will probably increase the time it takes you to fall asleep.

Why not try and use this insomnia curing programme as an opportunity (or excuse) to kick-start a healthy exercise programme at the same time?

Parasympathetic relaxation training and cortisol regulation

As we saw in Part 1, relaxation has an important place in an insomnia medicine chest. Insomnia and delayed sleep phase syndrome (DSPS) have been connected to an *out of phase* production of the stress hormone cortisol. As discussed in the introduction, for many people cortisol levels do not decline as they should towards the end of the day, but remain elevated because they over-produce stress responses that continue to stimulate cortisol production. When you lose the natural rise and fall of cortisol levels and they remain high in the evening it can interfere with your ability to sleep.

In Step 2 you will learn more about stress responses and how to permanently change the way they affect your body and sleep. For now, just start practising a daily parasympathetic relaxation response.

In Step 2 we will go into more detail about the mechanics of your internal stress responses, where they come from and what options you have to change them.

Meditation

Meditation is definitely worth learning if you have insomnia. Some meditations work better than others. See Appendix 5 for recommended meditations.

Melatonin

In addition to increasing your natural production of melatonin by controlling evening and night-time light pollution you can also take additional melatonin supplements (see Appendix 4 section for advice on choosing the right product). You do not need to take supplemental melatonin; however, if you want extra assistance to sleep better, supplemental melatonin is a healthy natural choice. If you choose to use melatonin supplements I recommend reserving them for either Step 4 of the insomnia programme, when we really restart better sleeping or, if you're on sleeping pills, reserve melatonin supplements for Step 5 as a more natural and healthy alternative when you start to withdraw from sleeping pills.

Bright light and darkness as sleep aids

The next two things in the insomnia medicine remedy chest are bright light therapy and darkness control techniques.

To recap what you learned in Part 1, bright light therapy early in the day helps insomnia; think of it making you more awake in the morning so that you feel more sleepy in the evenings.

By working indoors and exposing your eyes to too little sunlight in the morning and throughout the day and using too much artificial light after the sun has gone down in the evening your brain may be not getting the information it needs to run healthy sleep cycles.

The cells in the eye that send signals to your biological clock about outside brightness and darkness respond almost exclusively to a narrow band of wavelengths of light (specifically blue/cyan coloured light) and we can make use of this understanding to intensify the strength of your internal physiology to wake us up in the morning and make us fall asleep in the evening.

Using bright blue light in the morning compensates for the lack of natural daylight we get by working indoors during the day and sends a very strong timing signal to your biological clock which coordinates when your body should wake up and fall asleep.

Blue light entering the eyes in the evening reduces/stops melatonin production and imposing virtual darkness in the evening initiates melatonin production.

Bright light therapy (BLT)

Bright light treatment has been shown to increase night-time melatonin production and help insomnia, so I added BLT to my insomnia cure and found it was a powerful addition. Combining lithium with BLT stimulates the healthy activity of the biological clock, waking us up more intensely in the morning and creating a greater pressure to fall asleep in the night. Adding vitamin B-12 to BLT increases the rate of the rise and fall of melatonin release. By using the right blue light we can produce these effects with a short treatment time of as little as ten minutes, depending on the device you use.

A high end BLT device can be fairly expensive, but if you are on a budget there are still options available. For an up-to-date review of bright light therapy devices and my recommendations see my website (www.the-sleep-solution.com).

Total darkness

Setting up total darkness in your bedroom to the point at which you can't see your hand in front of your face, even during the day, stimulates maximum and sustained melatonin production throughout the night; this helps deepen and maintain sleep.

How to use darkness to treat insomnia

Once you've set up your light-tight bedroom all you have to do to reap the benefits of darkness is sleep in it! The only potential problem is if you leave your dark bedroom during the night, for a bathroom visit for example, and pass through any areas with sunshine streaming in through windows in the early hours of the morning or need to put the lights on to navigate your way around. The solution is to either put on some blue light-blocking glasses and/or install low blue lights everywhere you need them.

VIRTUAL DARKNESS

We will also take advantage of our biological clock's sensitivity to blue light only to improve our sleep. By excluding just the blue light from the artificial light you are exposed to in the evening you will still be able to read, use a computer, watch TV, eat your dinner, etc., but your biological clock will no longer receive any light signals from the outside and 'think' you are in complete darkness. Imposing virtual darkness for several hours before you intend to sleep will bring on an earlier and increased production of melatonin which increases sleep pressure when you need it.

Having initiated your melatonin production with virtual darkness you will maintain it with the total darkness you've created in your bedroom.

HOW TO USE VIRTUAL DARKNESS TO TREAT INSOMNIA

Impose virtual darkness on your eyes for at least two and ideally three to four hours before your bedtime. When blue light enters the eyes it imposes a clamp on the pineal gland, preventing it from making melatonin, but there is some delay between the lights effectively going out and the onset of a significant production of melatonin, hence you impose virtual darkness some hours before bedtime.

It only takes a brief exposure to bright light to diminish or shut down melatonin production for several hours and it's surprisingly easy to accidentally forget about the virtual darkness and expose yourself to bright light without wearing protective eyewear during the virtual darkness treatment. So I recommend starting to apply virtual darkness as soon as you can, to train yourself how to practise and maintain it. In the end, if you're serious about your health and maintaining great sleep, you'll want to get the yellow low-blue light bulbs.

In a relevant study (see Appendix 3) it was shown that a two-hour exposure prior to bedtime from self-luminous LED displays (tablet computers, iPads, etc.) can suppress melatonin production by 22 per cent; this is now a common experience for millions of people.

Combined together these light-reducing techniques enable you to exert a powerful positive effect on your natural sleep physiology. When you take sleeping pills you are adding potentially toxic artificial drugs to manipulate your physiology; with these light-controlling techniques you are adding natural forces (bright light and genuine darkness) to compensate for modern indoor living and naturally correct your physiology.

You should make a start on excluding light from your bedroom and reducing your evening exposure to light at this point in the insomnia programme. You will need to have a light-tight bedroom and at least a pair of blue light-blocking glasses to create virtual darkness before you can start the sleep inducing techniques in Step 4.

You should read Appendix 3 and start to take advantage of these techniques over the next couple of weeks, in readiness for Step 4 when you start to treat your insomnia.

Shopping list for the insomnia cure

I've specified the amount of pills you'll need for a month to get started, but for the whole two-month programme you will need double this quantity.

- B-12 methylcobalamin only 1000 mcg (see Appendix 2 for brands).

- Lithinase (lithium) (available from www.iherb.com).

- B-50 complex. You will need 60 pills per month. Recommended brands are Solgar, Now, Source Naturals. Vitamin B complex accentuates the effects of all the other remedies below and helps balance the nervous system when under stress. Two particularly interesting B complex formulas for our purposes are

Megasorb B-Complex by Solgar, which contains other useful micro-ingredients, and Higher Natures True Food B complex, which contains a lower dosage but is more far more absorbable and less likely to cause excessively vivid dreaming.

- L-tryptophan. You will need 60–90 pills per month. (L-tryptophan is available again for sale in the UK; however at the time of writing it is quite expensive so I buy mine from www.iherb.com in the US.) Now Foods and Source Natural are the brands I recommend, however an ideal sleep formula is Doctors Best, Best L-tryptophan enhanced with vit B-6 and niacinamide. The inclusion of a small amount of B-6 and niacinamide within this formula will increase the conversion of the tryptophan into the serotonin and melatonin that helps sleep; it is, however, 50 per cent more expensive.

- Magnesium. You will need enough pills to give you 400–600 mg magnesium a day for two months. A petite person needs 400 mg, a larger person needs 600 mg. Recommended brands are Solgar, Veridian, Now Foods. Magnesium citrate can be easily bought in health stores. A petite person should take 400 mg and a larger person should take 600 mg per day. These quantities relate to the amount of actual magnesium contained within the magnesium citrate; don't get confused with the total amount of magnesium citrate which will be a larger quantity. These days the amount of elemental magnesium delivered should be clearly stated on the label.

- Zinc. When not properly formulated zinc is hard to absorb so choose a good quality product. See further on in the book for advice.

- GABA. You will need 120–180 capsules. Recommended brand: Now Foods 500 mg GABA capsules. The recommended dosage is 500 mg all the way up to 6000 mg, with 2000–3000 mg being an average starting dose.

- L-theanine 100–200 mg. You will need 60 200mg tablets. Recommended brands: Lamberts, Now Foods, Source Naturals.

- Blue light-blocking glasses and/or yellow light bulbs, discussed above.

- A blue light box, see Appendix 1.

Remember, none of these remedies are addictive or have undesirable side-effects and you only need to take them for a few weeks duration to get things started. Once you've established good quality sleep you can then stop taking the remedies or carry on as you want to; if you do decide to stop, gradually reduce the dosage over a couple of weeks before eventually stopping. Having said that, I actually recommend people who are interested in maintaining optimal health to take magnesium and zinc supplements daily on a continuous basis because the level of these two minerals in our food has declined as a consequence of intensive farming. It's early days but research suggests supplementing B-12 may reduce brain ageing (Tangnay *et al.* 2011; Smith *et al.* 2010). A low dose of lithium extends lifespan. The tryptophan, GABA and theanine have no ongoing health benefits for people without insomnia, depression or anxiety.

Step 1: Mental exercises and recordings

Every day do a 25-minute relaxation by listening to the recording for Step 1, and perform one of the breathing exercises below.

Breathing exercises

The purpose of these breathing exercises is to train your system how to switch off stress responses and eradicate elevated night-time cortisol levels which disturb and prevent good sleep. You will learn more about night-time cortisol and sleep in the next chapter, for now please just start performing the exercises.

Below are two different breathing techniques you can use to help you overcome insomnia. The first technique, what I call parasympathetic breathing, involves slowing your breathing down, making long continuous deep and slow breaths; the second technique is called Buteyko breathing which involves very relaxed, minimal shallow breathing. Most people find they can do parasympathetic breathing and that it quickly induces a deeply relaxed condition; however, a small number of people find that when they do this long deep breathing they start to over-breathe and feel very uncomfortable, perhaps even stressed and panicky – the exact opposite of what we're trying to achieve. People that find parasympathetic breathing makes them feel uncomfortable should use the Buteyko method instead and should find it quickly calms the nervous system. The Buteyko breathing method is also a useful treatment for sleep apnoea and asthma.

If you've had panic attacks or asthma in the past it may be a good idea to learn the Buteyko method first before trying the parasympathetic breathing method. This way if you are one of the few people that experiences uncomfortable and stressful feelings and physiological reactions doing parasympathetic breathing you will be able to quickly antidote the uncomfortable stress responses by switching to the Buteyko breathing method which uses opposite techniques. On the other hand if you feel fairly confident that you'll be able to do slow breathing without problems, use this method. Proponents of both the slow yoga style parasympathetic breathing and the Buteyko techniques will insist that their method is superior, but it makes no difference which method you use as long as it fulfils the goal of inducing a calming feeling and therefore switching your internal physiology from a stress response to the relaxation response.

Do an absolute minimum of two 10-minute or one 15-minute sessions per day, but ideally do two 15-minute or one 25-minute session today. You may be interested to know that doing a 25-minute per day meditation (and these are breathing meditation techniques) has been shown to increase immunity by up to 30 per cent within three months. I believe this impressive effect is probably due to the reduction in the production of the stress hormone cortisol which when over-produced leads to a weakening of the immune system.

Parasympathetic breathing techniques
METHOD 1

- Sit in a comfortable upright position with a straight spine, either on the edge of a chair or on the floor with legs crossed.

- You may have your eyes open or closed but you must relax and defocus the eyes, perhaps allowing the eyelids to naturally settle three-quarters closed.

- Change the focus of your awareness so that you start to become more aware of yourself, your body and your breathing and less aware of the outside world, the stresses and strains of the day.

- As you change your focus from the external world to your own personal internal world become aware of the sensations of your breathing, notice the sensations of the breath entering your body, causing your belly and chest to expand, and then exhaling, causing your chest and belly to subside. You may also notice the sounds or sensations of the breath moving through your nose at the back of your throat.

As your focus shifts to your inner space, deliberately create a positive mental attitude even if it is contrived and artificial; you only have to fake it temporarily and your automatic nervous system will still respond. Try imagining internally smiling just with your eyes so that your eye muscles soften and relax; at first smile in general and then smile at yourself.

In the beginning completing the above steps may take you several minutes; with practice, however, you will be able to make all the above happen in less than a minute.

• Now start to change the speed and the length of your breathing so that you make each breath longer and slower. If it helps you can imagine that you're actually slowing down time. You do not need to exert much force or effort to change the breathing, instead do it in a very relaxed and relaxing way.

• To increase the parasympathetic relaxation effects deliberately make your out-breath even longer and even slower than your in-breath; long slow deep exhalations exert a powerful physiological effect, activating the parasympathetic nervous system, which cancels all previous stress responses within the body.

• Continue in this fashion: focusing your awareness internally, adopting a positive mental attitude, smiling with your eyes and breathing slowly for as many minutes as you can. When you lose your focus (as you inevitably will) and find your mind has drifted back to an awareness of the external world, simply open your eyes, take a sigh, even stretch and adjust your position if you want to, and start again from the beginning.

Most people find their ability to stay longer in the meditative state improves quite rapidly, but remember this is not a competitive exercise and being frustrated at your performance will only add stress into your nervous system and actually impede the benefits. The correct mental attitude to adopt is one of gentle perseverance; a subtle but definitive difference between meditation and deep relaxation is that during deep relaxation one adopts as passive and mental attitude as one possibly can, compared to meditation where one has to apply some effort to hold one's focus on the meditation, albeit gently applied.

Once you have mastered this useful technique you will be able to use it and switch off stress responses quickly and efficiently throughout the day and improve many aspects of your health.

Method 2

- Sit as above with a clock in front of you about waist height, so that when you partially close your eyes you can comfortably stare at the clock. You need to use a clock with a second hand so that you can visually see the seconds ticking away.

- Start inhaling when the second hand is in the 12 o'clock position and continue to inhale until the second hand reaches the 10 o'clock position. You should have completed a fairly deep inhalation during those ten seconds.

- Now exhale in a controlled and measured way so that you have fully exhaled by the time the second hand reaches the 20 second position. This means that you have taken 20 seconds to complete one breath and fully inhaling and fully exhaling.

- Start with the second hand at 20 past, inhaling again for 10 seconds to half past then start exhaling to 20 to, then start inhaling again until 10 seconds to, and finally exhale back to the 12 o'clock position.

- In other words you inhale for 10 seconds and exhale for 10 seconds, and inhale for 10 seconds and exhale for 10 seconds continuously, making each breath last 20 seconds and therefore taking three breaths in a minute.

- Continue in this fashion for 5–10 minutes, whatever feels appropriate, then slow the breathing down again, this time inhaling for 15 seconds (from 12 o'clock to quarter past) and exhaling for 15 seconds (from quarter past to half past), then inhaling for 15 seconds (from half past to quarter to). This makes a single breath last 30 seconds giving rise to two breaths per minute.

- Continue in this fashion for 5–10 minutes, whatever feels appropriate, then give up the clock watching altogether and continue for the last 5–10 minutes breathing freehand, slowing down your breathing in the slowest but most relaxed and natural breathing rhythm you can achieve without becoming out of breath or needing to strain.

- Spend 15–25 minutes per day performing this pleasant breathing meditation and you will improve your health tremendously.

Buteyko breathing technique

In the yoga breathing above you use your breathing muscles to take deep breaths, Buteyko breathing, on the other hand, is reducing one's breathing in a relaxed way taking diminished diminutive breaths.

- Sit in a comfortable upright position with a straight spine, either on the edge of a chair or on the floor with legs crossed. It is very important that you don't slouch forward so that your chest does not sit heavily down on your stomach.

- You may have your eyes open or closed but you must relax and defocus the eyes, perhaps allowing the eyelids to naturally settle three-quarters closed.

- Breathe only through your nose with your mouth closed at all times.

- Take two, maybe three, *very small breaths* breathing into your belly only and not breathing into your chest at all.

- Now gently hold your breath out (for the control pause) telling yourself relax, relax, relax, making your neck and your shoulders and your face as relaxed as possible. Continue holding the breath out until you feel the first twinge of needing to inhale again and then just let your breath go and then breathe normally, taking small breaths for about 2– 3 minutes or so before repeating the process of holding the breath out for as long as feels natural and comfortable. The sensation to breathe again could be just a slight twinge in your throat or diaphragm; look out for the signal and don't hold your breath a moment longer, so that you are absolutely positively not straining or stressing yourself at all. If you feel any stress or strain or you find that you have to take several deep breaths after holding your breath to get enough oxygen then you're pushing yourself too hard and *must* hold your breath for a *shorter time*. If you find it helps you can keep your head slightly backwards as you are doing the control pause breath hold.

• Continue breathing in this fashion and once you feel your system calming down start to also simultaneously change the focus of your awareness so that you start to become more aware of your body relaxing and less aware of the outside world, the stresses and strains of the day.

• As you change your focus from the external world to your own personal internal world become aware of the sensations of relaxation, peace and tranquillity as you continue this exercise.

• Now that you have shifted your attention from the outside world to your inside world deliberately create a positive mental attitude temporarily for the duration of the exercise, even if this seems contrived and artificial. The way I do this is to imagine internally smiling and smiling just with my eyes so that my eye muscles soften and relax.

• Spend about 8–12 minutes doing this exercise twice during the day and again when you get into bed to sleep. Each session would go something like this:

1. Spend 1–2 minutes gradually relaxing and slowing your system down, reducing and minimising your breathing.

2. Perform your first control pause (perhaps 15–30 seconds).

3. Rest and breathe in a relaxed way (2–3 minutes).

4. Perform a second control pause breath hold again, until you feel the need to breathe.

5. Then rest and breathe in a relaxed way for 2–3 minutes.

6. Then perform a third and final control pause before finally

7. Taking a long rest of 3–5 minutes.

With practice in time you can become very adept at using the above steps to reduce feelings of stress and anxiety in your system. The above method is sufficient for the purposes of curing insomnia, but there are many books and training seminars available to teach you the Buteyko breathing method if you wish to further develop your abilities over six months or so.

MINI BUTEYKO FOR EVERYDAY SITUATIONS

Take small minimal breaths through your nose in the following sequence:

1. mini breath in–out pause and stopped breathing for a count of 1

2. mini breath in–out pause and stopped breathing for a count of 2

3. mini breath in–out pause and stopped breathing for a count of 3

4. mini breath in–out pause and stopped breathing for a count of 2

5. mini breath in–out pause and stopped breathing for a count of 1.

You can perform these mini Buteyko sessions for several minutes while doing other things at the same time.

Sleep recording 1

The subconscious mental exercise included in the first recording asks you to start with something general; you will simply picture and imagine yourself becoming a good sleeper in the not too distant future. We do this in Step 1 to sow a seed in your subconscious mind of the *concept* of yourself as a good sleeper, the opposite of how you probably see yourself at the moment, and we will build on that concept. It does not matter if at this point in time there are still other parts of your mind convinced that you'll never sleep well again. We will build a different set of beliefs, eventually becoming what your mind experiences (sees, feels, believes) in the foreground. Your subconscious mind can be programmed just like everybody else's through repetition; all you have to do is engage in the exercises.

Summary of Step 1

In this first step you will prepare and set up everything you need for the insomnia treatment to come, order the remedies and make your sleeping area totally light tight. You will also make a start on training your nervous system how to switch off stress responses and lower the stress hormone cortisol with relaxation and breathing techniques. In this step you will also be introduced to the various natural sleep remedies that you will use throughout this book. Lastly you will keep a record of how well you are currently sleeping that we can use in the future to gauge your progress.

Eliminating Sleep Inhibiters, Understanding how Diet and Stress Responses Affect Your Sleep

Your goals in Step 2

1. Learn about all the things that inhibit good sleep and eliminate them. This list includes environmental influences such as bright light, stimulating TV, caffeine, heat in the bed, and internal influences within your own body (stress responses, cortisol).

2. Understand the how and why of parasympathetic relaxation training to deepen your practice.

3. Perform exercises to reduce stress.

4. Programme your subconscious to diminish and eradicate negative attitudes towards sleep and break the hold these have over you.

Eliminate sleep blockers

Start this week, and continue throughout the programme, eliminating sleep blockers in your diet, environment and internal physiology. Some of the things below may seem obvious, like avoiding caffeine, but please still abide by them; imagine each technique is worth a few percentage points and combined together with all the other techniques you are going to use they help you establish an overwhelming sleep pressure to knock out your insomnia. Everything from clean comfortable sheets to the right background noise can influence how well you sleep but let's begin this section with techniques you can use to affect the production and timing of two influential sleep-regulating hormones: melatonin and cortisol.

Bright evening light

Begin with simply dimming down the brightness of your computer monitors, TVs, living room lights, etc. In the living room this may be fairly easy to achieve; a trickier problem is that even a short burst of bright light, as may occur in the bathroom when we brush our teeth or remove make-up, or wander in and out of our brightly lit kitchens, can be sufficient to delay and diminish melatonin production for hours.

In Step 4 we will begin the insomnia programme treatments and you must be able to start strictly imposing virtual darkness on your eyes by then, so continue perfecting virtual darkness techniques, eliminating and changing blue light pollution. Your eventual goal is to put yourself into virtual darkness for at least 2 but ideally 3–4 hours before you want to sleep, to give your internal physiology time to acknowledge the darkness and initiate melatonin production.

Elevated evening cortisol

In order to fall asleep our bodies go through a series of winding down steps that need to occur for a good night's sleep; this winding down activity does not occur properly when we maintain stress responses. In this chapter you will learn about what happens inside your body when you respond to stress, what triggers a stress response and, most importantly, what you can do to stop your body over-producing stress responses so that cortisol levels can fall and your body can wind down and fall asleep.

Isn't there a pill to reduce cortisol?

You might be tempted to search for an alternative way of reducing night-time cortisol that doesn't require as much time and effort as training your system how to switch on the relaxation response. The search online will show that an evening dose of phosphatidylserine is reputedly a means of reducing high levels of evening cortisol and facilitating healthy sleep. My personal experience with this substance was that it would produce a brief, quite mild but noticeable wave of tiredness and inclination to sleep which some people may find useful. However, for me, phosphatidylserine produces a very undesirable and unexpected side-effect. Phosphatidylserine is recommended as a supplement to enhance memory and help offset age related cognitive decline; personally however I found it did the exact opposite! For several days after taking it my memory recall was significantly disrupted. For example I would find myself saying things like 'You know the thing you walk on, the bit on the side of the road, you know the whatchamacallit…the err, the pavement! This memory disruption occurred consistently after trying phosphatidylserine several times over a decade. If anyone can suggest a physiological explanation for this effect, or has had similar experiences please e-mail me (see Contact Details and Getting the Free Recordings).

If you're still interested the dosage of phosphatidylserine needed to lower cortisol is quite high, at least 600 mg and ideally double that, 1200 mg. Phosphatidylserine is expensive and is not a permanent solution to over-producing evening cortisol. I do not recommend it.

A much better approach is training your brain and nervous system how to quickly and efficiently switch on the parasympathetic relaxation response. This is a superior approach, not just because unlike phosphatidylserine relaxation training is completely cost and side-effect free but, more importantly, because once you have learned this skill you retain the ability and receive lifelong the benefits of normalised cortisol levels.

I've understood the medical value of reducing excessive stress responses for a variety of health concerns for over two decades now and I've looked at various means to achieve it. The only really effective technique I have come across to significantly change the way your system deals with stress responses is a three-month training programme of whole body relaxation. Many people believe that meditation will produce the same therapeutic effects, however I can tell you with some certainty that meditation does not produce the same therapeutic effects as lying on your back and training your body how to switch on a parasympathetic relaxation response (PRR).

For long-term health, and especially for an increased sense of well-being, doing a daily meditation is generally superior to doing PRR training. However, to significantly and permanently change the way stress in your mind influences your physical body PRR training is superior by far. I've seen people who were long-term meditators yet had a poor ability to switch off their stress responses and achieve deep relaxation. These long-term meditators seemed able to transfer their meditation skills and quickly pick up and learn the PRR, but it wasn't something that their system was naturally doing until they had undergone a PRR training programme.

In meditation one generally is sitting in an upright position and holding a certain mental focus, both of which maintains a higher level of tension (sympathetic activity) within the nervous system than lying down, systematically relaxing all your muscles and adopting a passive mental attitude.

What is a stress response and what causes us to produce them?

Stress responses versus feeling stressed

What's the difference between a stress response and feeling stressed? Many people think being stressed is an unpleasant *mental feeling* of being threatened or under pressure but this is not the same thing as your *internal physiology* producing a stress response in the background. For example, when you watch an exciting thriller or exhilarating sport you wouldn't say you *felt* stressed, because it was a pleasurable and exciting experience; however, your body responds to the stimulation and produces a stress response. This enjoyable stress response produces all the same physical changes as an unpleasant stressful experience. Actually short-term stress responses have been shown to improve health, so if you can switch off your stress responses quickly and efficiently stress can be good for you! The problem is when we produce too many stress responses and take too long to switch them off. The important point is just because you don't feel or think you are stressed doesn't mean to say that you're not triggering internal stress responses.

If the fire alarm at your workplace or in a cinema went off your nervous system would respond automatically and change your internal physiology to increase your chances of survival in a potentially threatening situation. Your heart and breathing rates, for example, would increase automatically without you having to tell them to do this and you probably wouldn't even be aware that these things were happening. Unless your heartbeat gets extremely high you don't notice it changing. If your heartbeat is 70 now as you're reading this but earlier today it rose to 85 because you were late for work, and your blood pressure rose accordingly, you would not have been aware of the internal stress response taking place.

During stress our body increases blood pressure, pulse rate, the intestines are clamped, blood is diverted away from the internal organs and more sent to the brain and muscles and the level of stress hormones adrenaline and cortisol increases; when you switch on the relaxation response our body responds by doing the opposite and decreasing blood pressure, pulse rate and the level of stress hormones. We can deliberately switch on our relaxation responses by temporarily deliberately changing our breathing, the tension in our muscles and stressful thoughts in our minds. Simply by taking conscious control of these things you can switch on the relaxation response in your body.

Stress responses happen automatically

A stress response is another name for the fight-or-flight response and refers to all the physical changes that occur inside our bodies whenever our mind perceives what it thinks is a potential threat. Even when the situation isn't really potentially dangerous, and our conscious rational mind can see this, the subconscious brain still produces stress responses every time it *perceives* something as a potential threat.

There is a region in the brain called the amygdala which makes connections between events in the outside world and potential danger. The classic example is a 'caveman' family walking through the woods as a twig snapped in the bushes and a lion jumps out and kills someone; the amygdala in the survivors will learn that the sound of a twig snapping in the bushes equals serious danger and it will produce a stress response. This same primitive stress response exists in us modern humans so that if, for example, you meet someone at work who looks the same or wears the same perfume as a scary teacher or a bully from your schooldays who made you feel threatened your amygdala will recognise the similarity and produce a stress response. Technically what happens is our senses (visual, hearing, smell, etc.) feed their information to an area called the thalamus which then assembles two reports based on the information it receives: a *brief summary* report is sent to the amygdala and the *full long report* is sent upwards into the higher conscious thinking areas of the brain. The amygdala scans the situation report, looking for signs of a match between the current situation and previous learned threats; when it finds a similarity it signals your nervous and hormonal systems to produce a stress response, ranging from a slight increase in heart rate and blood pressure through to a debilitating panic attack. The hormonal route is called the HPA-axis (hypothalamic pituitary adrenal axis) (see Figure 3.1).

The amygdala receives its brief 'bullet-point' report in half the time (12 milliseconds (ms) as opposed to 24 ms) that it takes for the more conscious thinking parts of the brain to receive and process the information; this means to say that the amygdala gets a first look at the world around you and the opportunity to decide this situation is threatening and stressful *before* your conscious brain is even aware of what is going on. So we are physically incapable of telling our brains not to produce a stress response, as by the time we've understood what is going on around us, and thought about it, it is too late and the amygdala will already have produced a stress response if it detects a match with a previously learned threat. The good news is that the amygdala can be reprogrammed and retrained so that it no longer makes the unwanted stress associations. Amygdala retraining is something I do in my practice using cognitive hypnotherapy and NLP and is beyond the scope of this book.

Briefly it involves putting the body and mind into a deep state of relaxation, then, whilst maintaining the relaxation response, connecting to the original memories and associations the amygdala uses to trigger unwanted stress responses and altering the memories, so that the amygdala no longer continues to make the unwanted stress connections; this is possible because it turns out our memories are not fixed in stone but are 'plastic' and malleable. We continue remodelling the memories until you are sure it feels different and then consolidating the amended memory in a way that your subconscious brain starts to automatically access the altered memories and no longer produces the unwanted conditioned stress responses.

Some people are put off this type of approach because they fear remembering the original dramatic stressful event, which is a great shame because, far from being stressful, the process immediately *diminishes* stress. It is also possible to work and process the painful experiences in what is called a disassociated condition where you are processing the problem from what feels like a remote and great distance without it being traumatising.

Let's not forget that sometimes the stress response our body produces is appropriate and protective because there is a real threat in our environment; for example, if you were previously bitten by wild dog, seeing or hearing a similar dog would activate your sympathetic (stress) nervous system and no matter how much relaxation training you do not want to become so relaxed that you no longer produce appropriate protective stress responses.

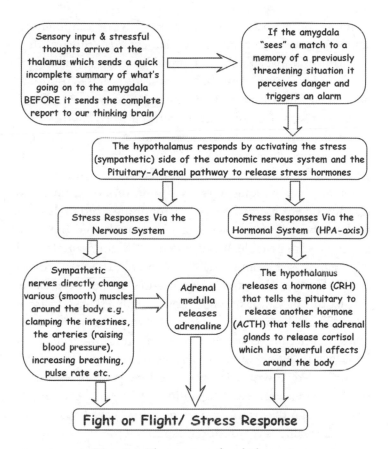

*Figure 3.1: The two routes by which stress in
the brain is conveyed to the body*

Sometimes, however, stress responses are switched on when there really is not any threat to our safety, for example in fear of public speaking and social anxiety. People vary considerably in their propensity to make and maintain stress responses. Some people have naturally very highly strung nervous systems, like a burglar alarm that is set too sensitively and is triggered just by a cat or strong wind. Layered on top of our genetic predisposition are our learned stress responses from our upbringing and from traumatic life events. In post-traumatic stress disorder (PTSD) to take an extreme example, sufferers often become highly sensitive to numerous, sometimes seemingly all, potential external threats; they may, for example, flinch and produce a strong full-blown stress response every time they hear a loud noise. You don't have to go through a war and be diagnosed with full PTSD to have stress-provoking memories and learned conditioning embedded in your subconscious brain that produces too many and too disproportionately strong stress responses for your health and happiness. I've also observed a considerable difference in how long it takes people to switch off stress responses. I've observed people maintaining a certain level of background stress from events that happened a long time ago; in people with irritable bowel system (IBS) for example (and I include myself as an ex-IBS sufferer) the IBS attack often occurs for five days after a significant stressful experience. At first this didn't make sense (how can a message sent from the brain to the bowels take five days to get there?) and yet relaxation training consistently adds significantly to helping IBS. Eventually I realised the problem was not how quickly or easily people with IBS were producing stress responses, the problem lay more in the ability to let it go afterwards, so that although they think they're okay and have let go of the stress the reality is that residual aspects of the stress response remain and maintain the stress response clamping effect on the intestines for days, retarding healthy movement through the intestines before finally culminating in an IBS attack. Long-term parasympathetic relaxation response training is the only effective therapy for nervous systems that have a propensity to hold on to stress.

If you feel you were brought up in a stressful or traumatic environment or believe you have been exposed to and stored significant stressful memories of threatening scenarios, or if you suffer from feelings of stress or have health problems that can be significantly worsened by stress, it would be a really good idea to undergo appropriate psychotherapy to change your subconscious programming and remodel stressful memories to stop them inappropriately triggering protective stress responses based on past traumas rather than current reality. It's not uncommon for people to find they are unable to perform the free relaxation training, because when they perform the exercise and quieten down their mind, rather than feeling relaxed they are troubled by painful and anxious feelings coming to the surface. The only effective solution I've found is to change and process the toxic and painful memories that are the problem. In the past I would have recommended long-term talking psychotherapies that would typically take a year or two to change painful memories sufficiently to allow one to proceed with the relaxation training; today, however, I would recommend hypnotherapy and NLP techniques which can access and remodel painful memories very quickly and efficiently in as little as four to six one-hour sessions and then allow you to proceed with the relaxation training. I still recommend analytical types of therapy for people who want to explore their feelings and find *meaning* in past events, but if you just want to stop painful memories producing unwanted and unhealthy stress responses and sufficiently lower your cortisol and stress responses use the faster therapy techniques.

When people attend my clinic for better sleep I often find there is one or more significant emotional events from the past contributing to the sleep problem by triggering unnecessary stress responses. Chronic insomnia (i.e. insomnia lasting more than six months) generally starts out as short-term acute insomnia induced by stressful life events. It may be that we do not have to look beyond the stressful events occurring at the start of the insomnia, however what made these stressful events sufficiently disturbing to cause insomnia is often due to earlier learned stress responses.

In another book on changing stress responses I'll explain remodelling stress responses in a lot more detail but all you need to know to cure your insomnia is how to prevent stress responses automatically occurring in the evening, activating your nerves and cortisol production to prevent you winding down and going to sleep.

There are three things you can do to change your learned and automatic stress responses:

1. You can complete the intensive training programme to teach your nervous system how to switch from a distressed condition into a deeply relaxed condition quickly and efficiently. Let me explain this: I watched a documentary on the television investigating which was the most stressful way to commute to work. The participants had a 24-hour blood pressure meter to monitor their level of stress and arousal and what happened to one of the participants is relevant; as this woman went into the Underground (subway) her blood pressure rose dangerously high without her feeling it, presumably because unbeknownst to her she (her amygdala) possesses a fear of something in the Underground (enclosed spaces, crowds, trains, fire, germs, etc.). What happened next is what we should concern ourselves with: it took more than six hours before her blood pressure gradually returned to normal, and as she did this twice a day, the consequences of her stress-induced hypertension could potentially take many years off her lifespan. If this woman did the parasympathetic relaxation response training you're about to do on this programme she would still produce the same stress response when she entered the Underground but she would get over it, switch it off and bring her blood pressure back down to normal in a fraction of the time, say 30–40 minutes or even much less if she really developed her skills. If you continue developing these skills with what I call parasympathetic breathing you can programme your body to automatically switch off minor stress responses throughout the day with a

few simple breaths that you can do at the same time as you do many everyday activities.

The parasympathetic relaxation response training does not stop you producing stress responses in the first place. However, it teaches you how to end and switch them off quickly.

2. You can use behavioural techniques to retrain the subconscious brain (amygdala and other areas) to no longer make a particular negative association that is harming rather than helping your health. For example a person may be able to overcome their fear of flying by repeatedly flying and showing their subconscious nothing bad happened. Even deeply ingrained beliefs programmed into the subconscious brain can be changed with the power of behavioural modification techniques; basically the subconscious brain and the amygdala learns through repetition; when you repeatedly see something going well/badly your subconscious brain starts to learn. We know from neuroscience that the expression you can't teach an old dog new tricks is actually wrong and our brains and memories have a plastic quality such that memories, especially simplistic associations like flying is scary, can be remodelled and reprogrammed endlessly. It's more analogous to a computer; you can install new software programs which overwrite the previous 'faulty' programs. We're going to use this phenomenon a lot on this insomnia curing programme; in Step 4 you change your bedroom behaviour in specific ways to overwrite the current programming in your subconscious brain which associates your bedroom with poor sleep and insomnia with a new programme which associates your bed with actually sleeping.

You may have had the experience of being sleepy in your living room and then by the time you've got ready for bed, brushed your teeth, switched the TV off, etc., gone to bed only to find that the feeling of sleepiness and desire to sleep has completely evaporated. What happens is your subconscious brain associates your bed with failing to sleep, which it perceives as a very stressful, potentially even threatening experience. You may, for example, lie in bed feeling anxious about how lack of sleep is going to negatively impact on your performance the following day, perhaps your subconscious mind even worries you could be fired or lose your promotion because of your poor performance. As you lie in bed awake thinking about all the negative consequences of sleep you are programming the primitive defensive parts of your brain like the amygdala to associate lying in bed with danger and negative consequences. As you prepare for bed, switching off the television, brushing your teeth and doing all the other steps that you need to do to get into bed the negative programming in your subconscious brain recognises you are about to do something stressful (try to sleep) and it activates a stress response, releasing cortisol and raising your level of arousal. Sadly your subconscious now perceives going to bed to sleep as so stressful it is literally trying to prevent you from falling asleep because falling asleep could be dangerous in a threatening situation. We need to completely change this and overwrite it with the exact opposite programming, so that as you start to prepare for bed your internal physiology starts to send you off to sleep.

3. The third practical way you can change your stress responses are hypnotherapy and NLP techniques. It

turns out that our mind can learn new things not only through behavioural modification but just rehearsing a scenario in our mind can help us to achieve it. For example, before performing a tricky manoeuvre like the high jump you will see athletes rehearsing the process in their mind. Modern cognitive hypnotherapy and NLP techniques to take advantage of this 'dress rehearsal in the mind' learning ability of the brain have been developed and advanced way beyond simple mental rehearsal. Let me give you a simple example. Sit comfortably and let your eyes close. Now imagine the most beautiful place you've ever seen. Picture it right in front of you, how does that make you feel? Now, in your mind, change the image in front of you, bring it up closer to you making it larger and larger, how does that make you feel? Now move the image away from you or yourself away from the image so that it diminishes in size, becoming smaller and smaller, how does that make you feel? Did the feelings you have about this beautiful scene change as you brought it up close to you and pushed it away from you? The feeling is probably intensified and then diminished. Next try bringing the image up to a pleasantly close and large position, now change the image as if it were a TV and you could control the colour and contrast, begin by intensifying the colour saturation and see how that feels and then drain the colour out completely, greying out the scene in front of you, now try diminishing the contrast so that the entire image fades out. I suggest you use your TV remote, go into the settings and see what it looks like to maximise the colour saturation then minimise the colour saturation, contrast, the brightness, etc. You could also probably change the way this beautiful scene made you feel by including other qualities such as what you can hear as you're immersed in the scene and then imagine turning the volume up, making the soundtrack louder or quieting it down and see how that changes how you feel. In NLP and hypnotherapy this phenomenon might be used in a way that changes connections your subconscious mind makes with your sleeping.

This is just one of the many modern therapy techniques to manipulate how you perceive your world. Throughout the insomnia treatment programme you will be performing mental exercises; some of the exercises you do in an active conscious way and others are read out to you during the relaxation training recordings.

The first technique above (parasympathetic relaxation training) teaches you how to switch off stress responses quickly and efficiently *after* they've already happened. The second technique (behavioural modification) reprogrammes the source of the stress responses in the first place, at least the stress responses you're having associated with insomnia, but it doesn't change the source of every stress response you have throughout the day. You might be tempted to think that if you could just switch off the stress response to that source you would never need to undergo the 50 hours of relaxation training but I can tell you from clinical experience that that just isn't the case. There are many reasons for this, including that some people have a more sensitive threshold than others with regard to provoking stress responses. The third technique above (reprogramming the subconscious mind) also changes the negative programming which produces stress responses in the first place but it enables you to programme things into your subconscious mind which you cannot do through behavioural techniques. For example, you could mentally practise inducing the feelings of being very sleepy and falling asleep, you could in your mind produce an image, a sound, a texture or feeling, even just a colour and shape which represents how your mind perceives good sleep, and then manipulate that as you did the beautiful scene above to induce and intensify feelings you're looking for.

In the recordings you are guided how to put yourself into a deeply relaxed trance-like state and then in that deeply relaxed state you perform mental exercises and rehearsals. Combining these two things increases the effectiveness of each technique, for example you could mentally practise rehearsing a scenario like going to bed which is currently producing unwanted stress responses and imagine remaining calm and relaxed as you do it, but doing this *at the same time* as being in a profoundly relaxed state intensifies the learning experience and anchors the association much more effectively. Once you've been through this process you can actually use these techniques for other problems where stress responses are producing a negative effect. You could prepare for an interview or a presentation by introducing a deep relaxation response then whilst maintaining the relaxation watch a mini movie of yourself going through all the steps involved in this stressful scenario. When you come to do the real thing you'll find with enough preparation you can take the edge off the negative effect of your nerves.

Training your brain how to switch on the parasympathetic relaxation response

All you have to do to train your parasympathetic relaxation response throughout the insomnia programme is listen to the recording and follow the instructions. You can continue using one of the recordings to complete your 100 days training or if you prefer once you have established good sleep you can complete your 100 days training in silence using the instructions available on my websites (see Contact Details and Getting the Free Recordings).

Objectives of the training

Remember that the point to doing all of this is to stop internal stress responses maintaining an elevated level of cortisol in the evening which activates your system and prevents you from being able to sleep. If you can perform the relaxation response training all well and good, but if you find you are unable to complete it because even just trying to perform it produces feelings of stress and anxiety then you'll need to use psychological techniques (hypnotherapy/NLP) first to remodel the original source of the stress responses before undergoing the parasympathetic relaxation response training.

With this training programme your brain will learn how to switch off the stress response in your system and activate the opposite condition, the relaxation response. In order to overcome insomnia and prevent its return three months of PRR training should be enough.

If you complete this full training programme it will *permanently* change the way your body responds after stress. Once you've trained your brain and nervous system how to do something like ride a bicycle or swim it never completely forgets that ability, so once you've trained your nervous system how to switch on the parasympathetic relaxation response with this programme you'll keep what you've learned for life.

The training is very simple: you will lie down once a day and combine several techniques that switch off stress responses and switch on the opposite, a state of very deep relaxation. During each of the steps on the insomnia programme all you have to do to train your brain and nervous system how to change your internal physiology from producing a stress response to a relaxation response is lie on your back and follow the instructions on the recording for that section. The recording will guide you through the steps of the relaxation technique then guide you through some mental exercises to help you sleep. It takes 100 days of training to permanently install the technique into your subconscious brain so that elevated evening cortisol and stress responses will never again be strong enough to lead to long-term insomnia. This means you will continue doing a daily PRR session for several weeks after you are already sleeping better. At this point you can continue using the recordings to guide you through the session or you can continue on your own in silence using the instructions available free on my website (www.the-sleep-solution.com).

This technique will teach your nervous system how to get into a deeper state of relaxation than you ever achieve in normal daily life and how to switch quickly from a stressed (possibly normal) state to a profoundly relaxed state much more quickly and easily than you have ever done before.

Where to practise

In the beginning you should find a quiet peaceful place for your practice; your bedroom is usually a good choice. For people without insomnia I often recommend lying on the bedroom floor because for them when they lie in bed they associate it with falling asleep and may actually find it harder-going learning to relax rather than to fall asleep. However, when you have insomnia it's probably useful to do the relaxation training shortly before the time you go to bed or even when you actually get into bed to sleep. Eventually you can learn to switch on the relaxation response almost anywhere, even in the middle of a busy and noisy environment, but for now do it in a quiet place.

Relaxation versus sleep and when to practise

People with insomnia and a sleep debt invariably nod off when they perform a deep relaxation. If this happens it's okay, your subconscious mind will still hear the instructions and work with the exercise. Believe it or not when you no longer have a sleep debt you will find that you no longer fall asleep but instead drop into a state that feels like it's somewhere in between being awake and being asleep. When you can do this it is actually a powerful sign that you no longer have a sleep debt and are therefore getting enough restful sleep.

Another option is to do the relaxation training before 2 pm and if you fall asleep allow yourself to nap up to 50 minutes only. It is recommended that at least for the first week of Step 4, when you start treating your insomnia, you don't take any naps at all to make yourself feel as tired as possible later in the day.

In my opinion if you could choose any time of day to do the relaxation training I would recommend as soon after arriving back at home from work as you can; this would imply the association in your mind with arriving back home and going into a relaxed condition.

As I've said the deeply parasympathetic state and the sleep state are totally different; when you fall asleep you are no longer in the deep relaxation response, and to make the insomnia cure *permanent* you want do more than just get to sleep over the next few weeks, you want to make permanent changes to your autonomic nervous system that will protect you from ever getting chronic insomnia again.

Eventually what you're trying to achieve is a deeply *relaxed but awake* state; it has a distinctive feeling totally different from sleep that you should come to recognise and be able to 'level-off' in that condition without falling asleep. It has been shown that when we are in this deeply relaxed state some of our internal physiology changes in specific ways totally different to being asleep or being in a normal awake mode.

Posture

Lie on your back with your hands comfortably by your side or resting on your hips; if you put your hands on your belly or your chest they will move up and down as you breathe, this tends to make it harder to completely relax the arms and shoulders.

It's probably not a good idea to cross your legs at the ankles, strangely it can make it harder to relax the lower legs, but you can try it for yourself. It can be very comfortable, particularly for people with lower back issues, to put a few pillows behind the knees to bend the legs, so experiment as you want.

Have enough pillows under your head so that when you completely and utterly let go of all muscle tension in your jaw *your mouth doesn't fall open*. When your mouth falls open you start breathing through the mouth and this can feel uncomfortable and make it harder to relax the throat and mouth. You want to raise the head sufficient so that when you completely relax the jaw your lips still touch.

Feelings and sensations that tell you that you have switched on your relaxation response

HOT HANDS AND FEET

When the stress response is dominant blood is withdrawn from our extremities especially the hands so they become cold. When some people switch on their relaxation response they notice their hands and feet becoming warmer, perhaps even feeling hot.

GURGLING SOUNDS FROM YOUR INTESTINES

Muscles in the intestines clamp off segments of the intestines during stress responses. When you activate the relaxation response clamped muscles relax and intestinal movement starts again. The sudden un-clamping of intestinal spasms allows backed-up material to move onward and this can produce audible gurgling sounds. Hearing these sounds is a particularly good (but not essential) sign for anybody training their relaxation response to treat irritable bowel syndrome.

SLOWING DOWN OF YOUR HEART RATE

Some people, particularly those with high blood pressure, say they can feel their heart thumping; they may notice the sensation stopping as they successfully initiate the relaxation response.

In addition to the above you may notice an unusual heavy or floating feeling in your limbs. The feeling you get with the relaxation response is a distinctive feeling, perhaps something you have not felt before. Once you've got a sense of how it feels to be deeply and profoundly relaxed see if you can intensify the sensation by deepening each of the things that induce it:

- Relax the body even more deeply.

- Completely let go of stress and make your mind even more passive.

- Slow your breathing even more.

- Keep the mind absolutely still by focusing on your breathing or focus word.

See if you can do these things even more perfectly and increase the depth of the sensation of relaxation. Be patient, it may take some time to be able to do this at will. Practise every day until you can, and remember once you've perfected this skill you keep what you've learned for life.

How long to train for

To consolidate this skill will take a person with average abilities at least 8 weeks, and by 10–16 weeks nearly everyone can become fully competent at switching on their relaxation response. This may seem like a long time and I know it's popular today to want everything instantly, but mastering the ability to change your stress physiology at will is developing something truly skilled. Continue performing a daily relaxation response training for even after you have started sleeping better to prevent cortisol and stress responses causing insomnia ever again. Over the next few years if you ever have a bad night's sleep immediately put yourself back onto a week or two of daily relaxation training to refresh your abilities and nip the problem in the bud.

In the future I recommend you adopt a tactic of overkill and treat even a single bad night very aggressively. Don't hesitate to put yourself back on the tryptophan, theanine, magnesium, zinc, B-12 and B complex, get up early, do bright light therapy and only go to bed when you feel tired.

Once you've mastered the parasympathetic relaxation response so that it's second nature you can train your nervous system how to go into a parasympathetic state while performing everyday activities. You can achieve this with a technique I call *parasympathetic breathing*, for instructions see my website (www.the-sleep-solution.com).

Now we'll continue looking at other things that can hinder good sleeping.

Caffeine and sleep

Caffeine temporarily blocks the effect of adenosine, the chemical that builds up during the day making us sleepy. Caffeine is fully broken down and its effects are eliminated within four to six hours, so even drunk at mid-afternoon should have no sleep-disturbing effect whatsoever. Pregnant women and women on the contraceptive pill, however, may take twice as long as this to fully eliminate the effects of caffeine from the system and should therefore avoid caffeine altogether during the insomnia programme.

Another important thing to watch out for is hidden caffeine in soft drinks and medications; read the labels and unless it's an essential medication don't use the product or any other caffeine-containing food after 2 pm.

Alcohol and sleep

Alcohol can have a sedating effect on the brain that may help you to fall asleep, however this sedating effect actually reduces your ability to enter into deep sleep. Deep sleep occurs early during a night's sleep, when any alcohol consumed prior to going to sleep would still be affecting you. It is known from measuring electrical activity in the brain that during deep sleep brain activity is greatly increased; sedatives such as alcohol and sleeping pills prevent or reduce this increased brain activity inpeding deep sleep. Therefore, although you may find alcohol helps you to get off to sleep, it can significantly reduce the quality of your sleep especially the crucial deep sleep that occurs in the early stages. Lack of sufficient quality deep sleep has the biggest effect on creating a sleep debt and making us feel tired the next day.

Alcohol breaks down at a constant rate in the liver but exactly how long it takes to fully eliminate all alcohol consumed depends on a number of variables such as how much food you have consumed and your gender.

Generally you should be okay if you leave one hour for every unit of alcohol consumed. A pint of weak beer (4%) contains 2.3 units of alcohol and would therefore need 2.3 hours to be eliminated completely from the body, a pint of strong lager containing 3 units of alcohol would therefore have to be consumed at least three hours before going to bed and two pints of strong beer would take six hours to be fully eliminated from the body; a standard 175 ml glass of red or white wine contains around two units and a large 250 ml glass of wine around three units; a small 25 ml measure of spirits should contain one unit of alcohol. As you can see, a very small amount of alcohol early in the evening could conceivably be consumed without interfering with the quality of our sleep, however the amount of alcohol consumed in several beverages cannot be fully eliminated in time and will diminish our capacity to enter into deep sleep.

To be on the safe side you may consider *during the insomnia programme giving up alcohol altogether.*

Once you've cured your insomnia for several weeks you can reintroduce alcohol. If you want to have better quality sleep, however, only drink in moderation and stop drinking several hours before going to sleep. For example, if you had important meetings or exams and wanted to be at your best and get a good night's sleep it would be best not to consume any alcohol the evening before. If in the future you find yourself using alcohol to help you relax and fall asleep read it as a warning sign that your sleep processors may not be functioning in a healthy way and you may be on your way to developing insomnia again. You can repeat the entire insomnia cure programme; it still works even if you have done it before.

Marijuana and sleep

I've seen many patients who developed insomnia whenever they gave up marijuana. Deal with this problem in exactly the same way as you would deal with withdrawing from sleeping pills. Do every step of the insomnia programme properly and slowly, and gradually reduce the amount of marijuana you consume as the sleep programme gradually restores and repairs your natural healthy sleeping processes.

There are two primary active compounds in marijuana: cannabidiol (CBD) and tetrahydrocannabinol (THC). THC is a compound that gives one a feeling of being high, it speeds up thinking and in some people causes paranoid and anxious thinking; it does not help you sleep. CBD, on the other hand, has anti-anxiety and calming effects; it's also useful in pain management. Pain is one of the leading causes of insomnia and high CBD-containing marijuana could be a useful long-term pain and sleep management remedy. The pharmaceutical industry has done trials on CBD as both an anti-anxiety and pain medication.

If you're going to continue using marijuana but need to improve your sleep avoid the commercial 'skunk' common in the UK which has been bred to deliver the maximum amount of THC and thus give you the maximum high for your money. The laws keep changing and so at the time you are reading this, if it's legal to grow your own, you can buy high CBD-yielding seeds and within six months produce your own. As a health professional I cannot recommend inhaling smoke and would only recommend using one of those sophisticated vaporising and cooling systems or eating it.

Re-establishing good quality restful sleep after giving up marijuana is absolutely doable, just as it is after coming off sleeping pills. However, it has been my experience that it can take twice as long, maybe even longer, to do than in someone who wasn't using any drugs at all.

Nicotine and sleep

Although many people say that they find smoking relaxes them its effects on the brain are actually quite complex and nicotine actually makes it harder to fall sleep. Once you're a good sleeper you may be able to get away with having a cigarette in bed, but during the insomnia cure programme cut down your smoking and don't smoke for a few hours before going to sleep. I provide a quitting smoking programme at my clinic.

Diet and sleep
Foods to avoid

For a small percentage of people a substance called *tyramine*, naturally present in certain common foods, produces adverse reactions. In these people tyramine produces a stimulating effect that may contribute to insomnia and migraines. So just to be on the safe side during the insomnia programme you should avoid tyramine-containing foods. These are: bacon, ham, salami, cheese, aubergine (eggplant), sauerkraut, tomatoes, wine and spinach. Another food to avoid is monosodium glutamate (MSG) (often found in Chinese food and ready meals) which can provoke tension headaches in some people.

Eating late at night

A small carbohydrate snack such as a piece of toast, or a banana in a small bowl of porridge (oatmeal) should not present any problems with sleeping; a large meal, however, especially containing animal protein, inhibits deep sleep and will need at least 2½ hours to digest, so leave sufficient time for this to occur.

Fluids late at night

If getting up during the night to go to the bathroom disturbs your sleep leave 90 minutes between your last drink and going to bed to allow enough time for excess fluids to pass through you. You may be able to improve and overcome this problem with a programme of bladder control and pelvic floor exercises; men with this problem should investigate the possibility that they have a prostate issue. Incidentally natural remedies and healthy diet can reverse and prevent prostate disease (Blumenfeld *et al.* 2000; Buck *et al.* 1990; Clark *et al.* 1998; Itsipoulos *et al.* 2009; Kristal *et al.* 1999; Pollard and Wolter 2000).

What liquids you drink is also significant; you shouldn't be drinking tea and coffee because of the stimulating effects of the caffeine they contain but these beverages also have a diuretic effect, meaning that they stimulate the production of urine increasing the chances you'll have to get up in the night; alcohol does the same. You might think that plain water would be the ideal drink before retiring, however it is possible to improve plain water. By adding about ¼ to ⅓ fruit juice to plain water you facilitate its entry into the cells and tissues of the body from the blood, thereby increasing its hydrating affect and reducing the amount of temporary excess fluid in the blood, which would otherwise be eliminated by the kidneys and increase urine output. If you use apple or orange juice make sure they are organic because these juices are mass produced with heavy-handed use of pesticides; however, non-organic pineapple juice is acceptable and what I use. Isotonic sports drinks are designed to do the same, however they typically contain excess simple sugars and there are hardly any I could recommend.

The tryptophan in turkey myth

Contrary to popular belief, eating foods like turkey and bananas will not raise your levels of tryptophan, the amino acid that is converted into melatonin and can help us sleep. Just to set the record straight on this.

There is some misleading information online and in print that you can get a serotonin boost by consuming carbohydrates. Some of the original research on this was done with rats and it turns out that rodent brains respond differently to carbohydrates than ours. Subsequent studies in primates showed that to get any serotonin boost from carbohydrates you have to eat absolutely pure carbohydrate, basically unhealthy foods like soda drinks. It was found that if a carbohydrate food contains as little as 4 per cent protein then the serotonin-boosting effect does not occur.

Even plain rice and potatoes contain more than 4 per cent protein, so they will not on their own give you a serotonin boost. However, other research showed that consuming a little plain carbohydrate, such as rice or potato, at the same time as supplementing tryptophan does increase the entry of the tryptophan into the brain, despite the inherent protein content of the food. This effect was demonstrated in primates (monkeys) and almost definitely occurs in us humans. My personal experience is that if I take my tryptophan supplement with a small potato, spoon of rice or handful of raisins I can achieve the same serotonin-boosting effect with half my usual dose. This may sound like a good idea, but I don't recommend it because what you are doing is inducing a surge of insulin which helps the tryptophan enter the brain. You may only get a small surge of insulin from a small portion of carbs but on a healthy diet you want to completely stabilise your blood sugar and prevent *all* surges of insulin.

So the way to increase tryptophan levels in the brain to increase the production of serotonin and melatonin is to take tryptophan supplements on their own last thing at night. (For more on carbohydrates, see Wurtman and Fernstrom 1975; Wurtman *et al.* 2003.)

Lettuce and kiwifruit

The only foods I can recommend with practical sleep inducing effects are lettuce and kiwifruit. Lettuce contains endorphin-like substances that have a sleep-inducing and reputedly antidepressant effect. The quantities needed to produce these effects are quite high, a whole medium-sized lettuce, for example, and consumed half an hour before going to sleep. It's quite easy to eat this quantity in the form of lettuce soup; however, most recipes for lettuce soup include cheese which is potentially a tyramine containing food which may stimulate rather than sedate you. You can find cheese-free recipes on my sleep website (www.the-sleep-solution.com).

A small study (Lin *et al.* 2011) showed that consuming two kiwifruit one hour before bedtime improved total sleep time by an average of 14 per cent and the time taken to fall asleep decreased by almost 40 per cent. Weight for weight, kiwifruits are also rich in antioxidants, facilitating tissue repair throughout the night.

TV and sleep

TV can produce stress responses, so another thing not to 'consume' prior to bedtime is stimulating TV such as thrillers, scary movies, sports or anything else that may stimulate the sympathetic nervous system and provoke the release of cortisol into your bloodstream. Also consider if a documentary may be upsetting and therefore inappropriate viewing while you are training your system to wind down and fall asleep.

You may feel that your mind can handle stimulating or provocative TV programmes, but understand that your *body* will produce an automatic stress response even if you don't notice it, and to overcome insomnia you have to stop producing stress responses in the evening to make your physiology wind down and allow the sleep system to take over. So until you are cured only boring TV is allowed for several hours before sleep. TVs are also a considerable source of blue light pollution, reducing melatonin production, and you must wear virtual darkness glasses when watching TV for at least three hours before your bedtime when you start the insomnia treatment in Step 4.

Noise and sleep

The brain has an amazing ability to learn to ignore continuous background noise as long as it's not too extreme. Erratic and variable sounds on the other hand take us by surprise and the brain may treat them as a potential threat, waking us up and releasing adrenaline. Do everything you can to avoid variable sounds and wear earplugs if this is a problem.

Continuous background noise on the other hand can affect us in different ways. If you were happy growing up in a city with background traffic noise you might actually miss it and feel less secure in the quiet countryside; another example would be the sound of the ocean. You can find devices that generate background sounds (birdsong, ocean waves, white noise, etc.) that some people find helps them sleep. On the other hand if you grew up somewhere very quiet and now live in a city or next to the ocean try earplugs to reduce external noise.

The bottom line is there are no hard and fixed rules with regard to continuous background noise and sleep; if you sleep best with Dutch acid trance music playing in the background do it.

The condition of your bed and bed linen

Have you ever noticed that you sleep better the first couple of nights after fitting freshly washed soft bed linen? How about treating yourself to some new sheets and for the next few weeks changing your sheets every few days to get that super comfortable feeling.

Is your mattress comfortable? Do you have comfortable pillows? Basically take a good hard look at your bed and ask yourself the question, if you were sleeping in a five-star luxury hotel would you be happy if they provided you with the mattress and bed linen you're currently using at home. If you can't afford a whole new mattress consider a mattress topper.

Make your bed a super comfortable inviting place you would really like to sleep in.

Exercise and sleep

Exercise and physical activity increase adenosine levels, which helps you sleep so you should do a lot; however, vigorous exercise that increases your body temperature within a couple of hours before bedtime is a bad idea because it raises your core temperature and believe it or not it can take hours to eliminate the extra heat. The conventional wisdom is to simply avoid vigorous exercise in the evening when you are attempting to overcome insomnia but I would not ever want to discourage someone from exercising and it can be so hard to find the time when you have an office job. There is a simple way around the problem and that is to take a long cooling shower or bath sufficient to give you gooseflesh at some point after the exercise, ideally 90 minutes before you go to bed.

Bedroom temperature and sleep

Remember in order for you to fall asleep and stay asleep your core body temperature has to fall and so the temperature of the area you sleep in can make a big difference to how well you sleep. Research has shown that people sleep better when the air in their bedroom is on the cool side and their actual bed nice and warm. During the night your body temperature falls to its lowest point around three or four in the morning. If you find yourself waking up in the night about that time notice how you feel; it might be that you are waking up because you're too hot and need cooler bedcovers; alternatively you may have become too cold and need warmer covers. Experiment with different thicknesses of bedcovers to see what works best for you.

If you allow your bedroom to get very cold, as I do, you may feel the need to warm your bed up with hot water bottles or electric blankets so that you don't have to get into such a cold bed that it wakes you up like a cold shower. Don't overdo it, only put a little hot water into the bottles and definitely put the hot water bottles out of your bed when you get into it, otherwise they can cause you to overheat and wake up.

Step 2: Mental exercises and recordings
You can do this exercise as you lie in bed.

Putting the stresses of the day to bed

1. Go through your body one part at a time and do the progressive muscle relaxation you have been doing to teach yourself how to switch on the parasympathetic relaxation response.

2. Now, in your mind, remember the things you did throughout the day as if you were witnessing them on a movie screen in a cinema. Either move the movie screen away from you or imagine moving yourself back so that there's enough distance between you and the screen that you begin to feel somewhat detached from the movie; you definitely don't want to be sitting right at the front of the cinema practically immersed in a huge screen in front of you. As an experiment try different versions of this exercise. In one version you go through the day starting at the beginning of the day and progressing as it happened and in the other version you start at the end of the day with the things that you were just doing in the last few hours in the evening and work *backwards*, what were you doing before that, and then what happened before that, etc. Try these different versions on different days and see which one you find the most powerful at putting the stresses of the day to bed; it may feel strange but you might be surprised to find that working backwards through the day is more powerful, but we're all

different, so simply choose the version that works best for you.

3. You don't have to remember every little thing that happened, just allow your mind to recollect the emotionally significant or stressful events.

4. Remember the significant events in full colour and include all the sounds you heard, what you said, what position your body was in, where the other people were, how did it feel, etc. Replay the events of that day.

5. When you recollect the significant event focus on keeping your body completely relaxed and maintain a detached feeling, but just alter the distance between the screen and you, increasing the distance if you must to shrink the size of the screen and diminish any feelings of stress associated with the events. From your relaxed and detached position allow your mind to receive and integrate positive experiences from the day, including lessons that you could learn from things which at the time may not have felt very positive and, as you do this, accept and forgive yourself for any mistakes or imperfections in your behaviour which may have been causing you a lingering feeling of stress. Imagine that integrating the lessons you have learned today into your subconscious mind will help to lead you to better experiences in the future. And now that you have told your mind to take what is positive from the stresses you had throughout the day imagine letting go of the stresses by dimming down the colours on the screen so that they become greyed out. You can continue to do this, either wiping out or blacking out the screen completely; alternatively you can move yourself and the screen further and further apart, increasing the distance so that the size

of the screen and volume of the soundtrack move further and further into the distance until eventually you're no longer aware of them.

6. Now move on to another significant emotional event you had in the day and repeat the same process of remaining relaxed and detached, integrating anything positive you can from it and then consigning the rest into oblivion.

Actually there is no reason why you have to limit this exercise to just the past day; if you find it useful, keep going over the past month or even several years, picking out and dwelling upon the significant emotional events and releasing the stress you are carrying in relation to them.

Dealing with anger

Chronically harbouring long-term angry and resentful thoughts can often be a part of insomnia. If you're having a problem with angry thoughts ruminating in your mind and preventing you from sleeping the exercise can take the edge off your feelings of anger sufficiently to allow you to sleep. In the beginning it may feel like an impossible task to use this exercise to change your angry thoughts and you should expect it to take several weeks or more daily practice. I've recommended using this exercise to many people over the years and perhaps as little as one in four people actually gave it a go; unfortunately anger can be such a difficult emotion to process (face up to and let go of) that it is very common to experience strong psychological resistance to even trying this powerful exercise. You may be in an on-going dispute causing feelings of anger which will probably make doing this exercise extremely challenging, however taking breaks from the anger by performing this exercise can be very helpful. Sometimes we can become stuck harbouring anger without taking appropriate actions to confront and resolve the source of the problem, held back by our own fear. Actually this type of stress coupled with inaction is extremely bad for our health (if you are interested in this see Seligmans' book *Learned Optimism* (1998)). It's also not uncommon to become stuck and unable to let go of angry feelings because of a sense of injustice; we may have suffered at the hands of someone else and be reluctant to let the 'guilty' party off the hook without being made to pay or make recompense. Unfortunately we can become stuck in these positions holding on to feelings of anger for many years that primarily only hurt ourselves, including keep us awake and have little or no useful purpose. If this is your problem practice the technique below for 25 minutes per day for 100 consecutive days to stop anger harming your health.

This powerful mental exercise helps resolve anger in several ways. First it helps you to detach from and let go of the anger which you cannot control; second it helps you clarify and see clearly what actions you may be able to take to stop and get away from the source of your anger; third it calms your anger, which helps you to be more effective in whatever actions you may decide to take.

Exercise to stop anger keeping you awake

You may feel reluctance to engage in these exercises because it feels like you're enabling the perpetrator or person involved in the source of your anger to get away scot-free, but think of this exercise just as a mental trick to help *yourself* release toxic anger from your mind and sleep better.

This exercise takes about 15–20 minutes.

1. Sit comfortably in a peaceful place, ideally with a straight spine, and dwell on your angry feelings. Say inside your mind or even out loud but not shouting 'I feel angry' and accept that this is how you feel right now.

2. Make a slight smile with your mouth and imagine you are smiling with your eyes.

3. Change your breathing either to long slow breathing or the Buteyko breathing method, as you prefer.

4. Now you are going to generate and cultivate feelings of compassion, acceptance, kindness and generosity which antidote feelings of anger; first you generate these feelings for yourself for 5 minutes and then later you will do the same for the person or persons you have angry feelings about. To generate feelings of loving kindness you can mentally repeat or chant the following:

   ○ May you be well.

   ○ May you be happy.

   ○ May you be free from ills.

   ○ May you be free from suffering.

Think of this as a kind of positive blessing and try and generate feelings of kindness as you repeat it. You can imagine looking at yourself in front of you or even seeing yourself in the mirror as you say this to yourself. This step is about generating self-love, self-acceptance and forgiveness.

5. Now generate the same qualities of loving kindness you did in the previous step only this time you picture the person or situation that is the source of your anger in front of you and you direct feelings of loving kindness towards them. However difficult it may be, ask yourself how much longer do you want to live with this anger and is it now worth trying something radical to get rid of it. Again mentally repeat:

- ○ May you be well.

- ○ May you be happy.

- ○ May you be free from ills.

- ○ May you be free from suffering.

Generate feelings of loving kindness as you do this and wish them towards the person or situation that makes you feel angry for about five minutes.

6. Now imagine the person/situation that makes you angry in front of you once more. Admit to yourself: 'I feel angry', but now imagine the person doing or saying something quite unexpected, imagine them performing acts of kindness towards you in a genuine and concerted effort to apologise for what they have done that has made you so angry. Imagine if they could admit and explain the problems, weaknesses and flaws that they possess which make them behave the way they have. For this exercise to work you must imagine yourself receiving and accepting the kind things they do and say to apologise and make amends. You're not expected to do this exercise once and then completely forgive and forget the situation, just do the exercise and see if it changes your feelings.

7. Now raise these questions: what is my anger truly about and what actions if any I should take? Ask yourself:

- ○ What am I really angry about?

- ○ How shall I respond to this situation?

- ○ If the anger had a voice and I listened to what it is saying what is the angry feeling asking me to do?

- What is the first step I could take – great or small – that would lead me to becoming free of my feelings of anger?

N.B. Do not go out and take the action which came to your mind straight away; however right it feels now wait at least five days, repeating the exercise daily, continuing to calm your anger and also think through the consequences of the action that first came into your mind and whether or not this will lead to a positive outcome.

The previous steps should have calmed your anger from raw emotion to a clear and clean feeling about the situation. From this position of greater self-respect (Instruction 4) and diminished anger towards the perpetrator (Instructions 5 and 6) you can choose to take appropriate action or you may decide that the best action you can take is take no action at all. If you decide to take action work through this exercise many times until you have gained control over your anger and can remain calm in whatever action you take. What you want to be able to do is respond in a strong, calm and respectful manner rather than reacting from a position of anger and defensive instinct.

SUMMARY OF THE EXERCISE

- Sit comfortably and admit 'I feel angry'.

- Internally smile with your eyes and mouth almost invisibly. Relax.

- Calm your breathing.

- Generate feelings of acceptance, compassion and loving kindness towards yourself for five minutes. Now do the same thing but wishing those feelings towards the person at the centre of your anger for five minutes.

- Now imagine the person performing acts of kindness and contrition to apologise and compensate for the anger they have caused you.

- Now ask the question: what is the first step I could do to reduce my feelings of anger?

Some additional thoughts on anger

Ask yourself: does the anger I feel towards a particular person feel similar to or remind you of some previous situation and try just as a mental exercise telling yourself for a few days the anger you have towards the person involved is not fully appropriate because you are transferring and misdirecting previous feelings of anger onto the current situation. After a week of privately performing this mental exercise see if it shifts how you feel your position and if it does even slightly this tells you that at least some perhaps most of the anger you feel is misdirected anger and until you have worked on yourself you constantly remind yourself that what you feel in the current situation is disproportionate and you are not capable of taking appropriate action. You could combine the self-help exercise above with several sessions with an NLP practitioner to release and neutralise the anger you are holding from the past.

Another consideration is whether the anger derives from feelings of being threatened and if so what are you afraid of? Try another mental exercise for a week or so just as an exercise, tell yourself: I feel threatened by this situation because...? Or ask yourself what is the worst thing that could happen in your imagination and listen to any answer that comes into your mind no matter how farfetched. Now consider if the threat is really a problem or is unrealistic and only really exists inside your own mind. Just like misdirected and transferred anger the cause of inappropriate feelings of being threatened can have its origin in past experiences and you can quickly overcome these with a few therapy sessions.

In cognitive hypnotherapy and NLP we have two wonderful techniques for dealing with such situations. One technique, called Timeline reprocessing, enables you to mentally travel back in time through your life to revisit the first significant emotional event connected to your current feelings of anger (or any other problem for that matter) and then use various mental exercises to remodel your memories of the significant emotional event. Psychologists have shown that our memories are not fixed but rather they can be changed by being revisited and remodelled, by adding new information to them. This changes how we feel in two ways, first changing a memory changes whether or not our mind and our amygdala finds any similarity between the past and present; second Timeline therapy can change the *emotional connection* you have or make with this memory, so by revisiting a painful memory in a relaxed and empowered way that diminishes the pain you previously always felt this memory ineffectively alters the emotional connection and association your mind makes with this memory. This is not that hard to understand; if you are very upset by an experience and talk it through several times with your friends who lighten the atmosphere with some appropriate humour you might find yourself quite quickly getting over the original upset.

Another effective technique we use in NLP is called Parts Integration, where your mind is directed to focus inwards on inner conflicts and conflicted feelings and then discover for itself how to unite your conflicting parts by finding a deep understanding of how all the parts of you were actually united by underlying common values and your drive to avoid pain and move towards pleasure and happiness.

Sleep recording 2

It's very common for people to wake up momentarily at the end of a phase of rapid eye movement (REM) or dreaming sleep; a good sleeper would just turn over and go straight back to sleep; a poor sleeper system will overshoot so to speak, wake up fully and then find it hard to go back to sleep. In this recording we make adjustments to your subconscious to adjust the depths of your sleeping system so that you stop overshooting and waking up. These adjustments may fix the problem right away or you may find that it is only as you progress through the rest of the programme that this problem goes away.

Summary of Step 2

In this step you learned to eliminate many things from your external environment which reduce your ability to achieve good sleep and about how to change things in your internal physiology that hinder (cortisol) and help (melatonin) good sleep.

You learned about two significant techniques to improve your sleep: how to train your nervous system to permanently stop stress responses over-producing cortisol and how to stop light pollution in the evening blocking healthy sleep-inducing melatonin production.

You also learned mental exercises to put the stresses of the day to bed as you lie in bed falling asleep and how to stop anger keeping you awake. You can use either or both of these exercises.

These first two steps involved quite a lot of learning. There is less of that to do in the next step before we begin insomnia treatment proper.

~ Step 3 ~

Understanding Sleep and Health, Pre-loading Sleep Supplements

Your goals in Step 3

1. Learn about sleep and health to dispel any myths you may have about sleep that may add to your worries about sleeping.

2. Perform mental exercises to let go by clarifying your goals and programming your subconscious mind to figure out solutions to your problems while you dream.

3. Start taking the preparatory supplements.

4. Listen to the third recording, which includes an exercise of mentally rehearsing getting ready for bed and remaining asleep.

Step 3: Supplements

Start the following supplements to pre-load these sleep-influencing nutrients into your system before you start the BLT and sleep scheduling techniques in the next section.

Supplement dosages (take with food)

- B-50 complex: one with breakfast and ideally another with dinner. If you find that this much B complex gives you excessively vivid dreams that disturb your sleep omit the second evening dose. Vitamin B complex facilitates the effects of all the other remedies below and helps balance the nervous system when under stress. Take with meals.

- Magnesium: A petite person should take 400 mg and a larger person should take 600 mg per day. This is the amount of actual magnesium contained within the magnesium citrate, not the total amount of magnesium citrate. The amount of elemental magnesium delivered should be clearly stated on the label. Take with meals.

- Zinc: Take 30–50 mg with dinner or last thing at night if it doesn't give you a stomach upset. You could take half with dinner and half last thing. If you get the Food State zinc you only need 30 mg (two tablets) and will be able to take it last thing on an empty stomach without problems.

- B-12: 2000 mcg held under the tongue without swallowing for 3–6 minutes.

- Lithinase: 2 capsules before bed.

What happens when we sleep

This section is just for information, you don't have to memorise any of this.

As we go through the night we pass through several distinctive phases of sleep, during which the brain exhibits quite different and distinctive patterns of brainwaves. These distinct phases can be illustrated in what is called a sleep histogram (see Figure 3.2). First we become drowsy and begin to 'nod-off' briefly. We then cycle down in distinctive steps from light sleep through to deep sleep and then back up into a lighter form of sleep during which we do most of our dreaming called rapid eye movement or REM sleep. From REM sleep we may briefly momentarily wake up before cycling back down into deep sleep again. Averaged out each cycle lasts about 90 minutes so we will go through four or five such cycles per night before finally waking. Some people take too long to cycle down into deep sleep and can't complete enough sleep phase cycles to wake feeling refreshed; other people complete the initial deep sleep phases but then wake up too completely immediately after each REM dreaming phase and have difficulty going straight back to sleep again.

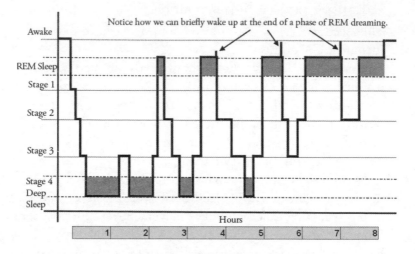

Figure 3.2 Sleep histogram

The two most important phases of sleep are deep sleep and REM sleep. For the sake of simplicity think of deep sleep as when the body gets its physical rest and REM sleep as when our mind integrates the experiences and things we've learned during the day to enrich our long-term memory and wisdom; this is the phase during which we figure things out and work out solutions to problems when we say 'will sleep on it'. Notice how we have the longest phases of deep sleep early in the night and that these become progressively shorter as the night goes on replaced by progressively longer REM phases. At the end of longer REM phases you may wake up momentarily; a healthy sleeper will just turn over and immediately go back to sleep and a poor sleeper may not be able to do this and become fully wide-awake at this point. Throughout this programme you will use remedies and do exercises to speed up your ability to get into deep sleep and to enhance your ability to return to sleep if you momentarily wake up after dreaming.

Stage one non-REM sleep (REM stands for rapid eye movement)

This is what happens as we begin to sleep, it is the classic 'drifting off' phase. It is characterised by: breathing becoming slower and more even, blood pressure falls, muscles relax and make little or no body movement apart from sometimes occasional jerking, blood flow to the brain is reduced and the actual temperature of the brain declines. This is not genuine sleep, it's more akin to relaxation and a prelude to entering sleep.

This phase lasts about ten minutes.

Stage two non-REM sleep

This is a deepening of stage one, whereby the sleeper gradually descends deeper into sleep, becoming progressively detached from the outside world and more difficult to awaken. Body functions gradually slow down, such as metabolism, heart output, blood pressure, etc.

This stage is in fact very light sleep but it's not uncommon for some people with insomnia to drift into this phase then wake up and fail to recognise that they were asleep. Many studies have shown that people who claim they do not sleep at all do in fact drift in and out of sleep without recognising it. This is not to say they don't have a sleep problem that needs treating, for they have not slept deeply enough to wake feeling fully refreshed. *An important part of overcoming insomnia is learning to recognise the sensations and experiences of falling and being asleep.*

This stage lasts about 20 minutes.

Stage three non-REM sleep

During this stage the electrical waves in the brain become slower and much larger. At this stage it becomes far more difficult to awaken the person compared to stages one or two – it takes a lot of noise or physical contact.

Stage four non-REM sleep

This is the deepest stage of sleep; the sleeper will be virtually oblivious to the outside world. Many bodily functions calm down to the deepest state possible of physical rest. If a person is awakened during this phase they may be confused, disorientated and unable to function normally for quite some time, experiencing a kind of 'sleep drunkenness'. Sleep walking and bedwetting begin during this phase. The first phase of stage four sleep is usually the deepest and lasts about 20–40 minutes, after this we revert back to the lighter stage three and two sleep before entering the REM sleep phase, when we dream for the first time.

Stage four deep sleep provides the brain and body with significant rest and renews our physical and mental energy. Loss or lack of stage four deep sleep is the most important in terms of tiredness and mental impairment the next day. Loss of the next stage of sleep REM, or dreaming sleep, more significantly impairs our ability to process and integrate what we did and learned the previous day.

REM sleep stage (when we do most of our dreaming)

When we enter the REM sleep phase the brain suddenly changes its activity, with brainwaves becoming much smaller and more frequent; we also get big bursts of rapid eye movement from side to side, hence the name rapid eye movement (REM) sleep. This is when we dream. Activity within the body perks up considerably during the REM sleep phase compared to the non-REM sleep phases, which are characterised by progressive relaxation. So for example blood pressure may increase drastically, breathing becomes irregular and oxygen consumption increases, the face, toes and fingers may go red, and blood flow to the genitals of both men and women is increased; however, the large muscles that move the legs and the arms for example are literally paralysed, so you may dream you are walking and moving around, but it's all in your mind, as your real muscles are disconnected and remain still.

The first period of REM sleep is usually short lived, as little as 1–10 minutes; subsequent REM phases become longer lasting 30–45 minutes, enabling long and complex dreaming. Throughout the rest of the night we cycle between REM and non-REM sleep another 4–6 times with each cycle lasting an average of 90 minutes.

The first two cycles of REM sleep are preceded by phases of long deep stage four sleep; as the night progresses phases of deep sleep become shorter then disappear and phases of dreaming REM sleep become longer.

In summary, in the beginning of the night we drop through lighter sleep stages down into a long deep non-dreaming sleep phase; this phase is very important to feeling rested the next day. We then come up into a lighter type of sleep when we dream briefly, before descending into another phase of deep sleep shorter than the first one. We continue cycling like this, spending less time in the deep sleep and more time in dreaming REM sleep, as the night progresses.

Dreaming REM sleep is actually quite a light level of sleep and it's quite normal to briefly wake up at the end of a REM sleep phase. A good sleeper will just roll over and go back to sleep straightaway without even remembering they woke up; a poor sleeper/insomniac, however, may wake up fully at the end of dreaming REM cycles and have difficulty going back to sleep. Since more deep sleep and less REM sleep occurs during the first half of the night most people will wake up during the second half of the night rather than the first.

Dreaming REM sleep is important for learning; studies have shown that when a person's REM sleep is prevented or disturbed they are less able to absorb and integrate what they have learned during the previous day.

One of the major limitations of sleeping pills is that they actually suppress *all* brain activity, including the brain activity that normally occurs in both deep and REM sleep, so although sleeping pills sedate you helping you to *fall* asleep your brain is prevented from entering into a deep REM sleep and you do not get restful sleep. This often causes people to feel sleepy the next day, not to mention the possibility that sleeping pills may increase mortality (see sleeping pills pages 183–5).

Sleep and health

How much sleep do we need?

The simple answer is there is no correct number of hours. The amount of sleep a person needs not only varies from individual to individual but varies according to your age. Some people appear to be able to survive on less than average amounts of sleep, but there is no medical test you can have to determine how much sleep you need, so the most reliable way to know how much sleep you need is simply to look for signs of sleep debt during the day, like yawning, etc. and if you demonstrate evidence of lack of sleep try improving your sleep to see if the signs go away.

As a guideline it is suggested that:

- Newborn infants up to 2 months need 12–18 hours' sleep per day.

- Infants 3–11 months need 14–15 hours.

- Toddlers 1–3 years need 12–14 hours.

- Pre-schoolers 3–5 years old need 11–13 hours.

- School-age 5–10 years old need 10–11 hours.

- Teens 10–17 years old need 8.5–9.5 hours.

- Adults need 7–9 hours.

Studies into the overall consequences of sleep deprivation have produced contradictory findings. Some studies appear to show little or no significant long-term negative effects on physical health from lack of sleep, however this seems at odds with many people's personal experience of lack of sleep; you may have experienced becoming ill and rundown following a period of insomnia, however both the rundown immune system *and* the insomnia could result from the concurrent stress you are experiencing, so it becomes harder to isolate the effects of lack of sleep from other issues going on in your life at the same time. Similarly a poor diet, high sugar and lack of exercise may contribute both to insomnia and to developing poor health but we cannot say it was the lack of sleep that was the cause of your problems.

What is not in doubt, however, is that lack of sleep has a direct, immediate and significant negative effect on your *mental* abilities. What is nice to know is that these effects are not permanent and full mental performance is quickly restored following adequate sleep.

So you may be pleased to know that if you have suffered from long-term insomnia the bulk of the evidence suggests that there will be no long-term physical or mental negative consequences once you cure your insomnia.

The popularly held belief that we need eight hours of sleep per night is wrong. A very large study in 2002 involving more than 1 million participants showed that people who sleep eight hours or more actually die younger than people who sleep 5–7 hours a night. Sleeping for less than five or more than eight hours per night was associated with reduced life expectancy.

Over the six-year period of the study people who slept eight hours or more were 12 per cent more likely to die than people who slept only seven hours per night. Occasional periods of insomnia were not found to be linked to higher death rates, but taking sleeping pills is associated with dying earlier, as we shall see later.

At this stage we must be very cautious about drawing conclusions from this type of study; for example, many of the people who slept more than eight hours were from low social and economic groups and unemployed, so there could be other explanations apart from oversleeping to account for the reduced life expectancy.

All the study has done however is observed an association between life expectancy and how much a person sleeps; this doesn't prove that how long you sleep affects how long you're going to live. So until we get further research we don't know if setting your alarm earlier and forcing yourself to only have six or seven hours of sleep as opposed to eight will make you live longer. One consideration I would suggest is important is that osteoporosis is on the rise and we know that when the body is inactive the bones slowly waste away and when the bones are put under stress through exercise they get stronger. We already spend far too many hours sitting down in offices to maintain good bone health and osteoporosis is on the rise, so if you are a very long sleeper or spend a lot of time in bed make sure you compensate for that by doing strenuous weight-bearing exercises such as strength training, rebounding and using vibration plates. If you are a night owl you may also be low on the vitamin D needed for healthy bones.

Can we recover sleep debt?

When deprived of deep sleep the body will spend more time in deep sleep the next time it can sleep and will try to recover 100 per cent of the missed deep sleep, compared to about half of lost REM sleep. People deprived of REM sleep or who have their REM sleep disrupted will fall into REM sleep as soon as they fall asleep, even during a quick nap.

You don't actually have to worry about sleep debt and you don't need to give yourself extra time to catch up because your body automatically makes all the necessary changes and adjustments to the length of time of the sleep stages the next time you sleep, so that you catch up automatically. The scientific evidence suggests that it's not possible to go

Monday to Friday sleeping too little and then completely recover all your mental and physical performance with a single good night's sleep (*ScienceDaily* 2007). Concentrate instead on just getting a good night sleep each night with the techniques in this book and once you are fully recovered allow yourself to occasionally use power naps in the first part of the day to compensate for feelings of tiredness and improve your performance. Remember if you're tempted to sleep in late during the weekends you may upset the timing of the 24-hour biological clock, and to prevent this happening you must wake up and give yourself a BLT session at the same regular time you do during the week.

Interestingly a study published in 2009 (Rupp *et al.*) suggested that if you know you're going to have a short night you can actually 'bank' some extra sleep in advance to offset subsequent tiredness.

Effects of lack of sleep and why we need to sleep

Surprisingly we still don't really know exactly why we have to sleep and discussing the scientific theories about why we need to sleep is beyond the scope of this book. What we do know is what happens to the body and mind when you don't get enough sleep.

- Lack of sleep causes daytime drowsiness and contributes to accidents, including fatal traffic accidents.

- Lack of sleep significantly impairs your mental abilities and performance including your memory, ability to learn, make decisions, etc. It also tends to make people feel very down and miserable.

- Lack of sleep is bad for your sex drive.

- Lack of sleep makes you look older. Sleep deprivation increases the body's production of the stress hormone cortisol. Long-term high levels of cortisol are not only bad for the immune system but they also age the skin. Lack of sleep also reduces the overall amount of growth hormone the body makes; growth hormone repairs and rejuvenates our skin, muscles and bones.

- Lack of sleep may contribute to weight gain.

- Lack of sleep (less than five hours per night) may increase your chances of developing Type II diabetes.

Many people with insomnia feel that condition must be doing them a tremendous amount of harm and it may help you to know that quite often lack of sleep does not cause any long-term damaging health effects, most of the effects of insomnia are reversible and, for most people, the worst consequence of insomnia is the fully reversible mental effects, how bad it makes you feel and the increased risk of having an accident. All the other effects of long-term insomnia can resolve themselves quickly and spontaneously as soon as you start sleeping well, however recovering from Type II diabetes and losing gained weight may take considerable effort.

Let's look at the consequences of lack of sleep in more detail

MENTAL EFFECTS OF LACK OF SLEEP

Without enough sleep our mental functioning and well-being decline significantly. The mental decline you experience with lack of sleep is probably the worst aspect of insomnia; the good news is it recovers completely and fairly quickly once you start to sleep better again.

IMPAIRED JUDGEMENT

In our increasingly fast-paced world, functioning on less sleep has become a kind of badge of honour, but there are very few people who genuinely thrive on just a few hours of sleep a night. Sleep-deprived people are prone to poor judgement when it comes to assessing what lack of sleep is doing to them. On the other hand, for some people with insomnia the way that lack of sleep can affect our interpretation of events causes them to underestimate how much sleep they are actually getting and overestimate the harm it is doing to them.

If you work in a profession where it's important to be able to judge your level of functioning, a reduced ability to make sound judgements can be a big problem.

INCREASED ACCIDENTS

Inquiries judge sleep deprivation to be a factor contributing to some of the biggest disasters in recent history: the 1979 nuclear accident at Three Mile Island, the massive Exxon Valdez oil spill, the 1986 nuclear meltdown at Chernobyl, for example, but daytime drowsiness due to lack of sleep loss is also a big everyday public health hazard, especially on our roads and in our hospitals where mistakes cost lives. Drowsiness can slow reaction time as much as driving drunk.

IMPAIRED LEARNING

Sleep plays a critical role in thinking and learning; lack of sleep impairs attention, concentration and problem solving. This makes it more difficult to learn new things efficiently.

To make matters worse, during REM sleep the brain produces what are called sharp wave ripples, which are responsible for consolidating and integrating what we have learned during the day into our long-term memory banks. If you miss out on REM sleep your ability to learn and remember what you learned and experienced during the day is impaired.

Depression

As well as the inevitable feelings of stress and unhappiness that insomnia can cause it is common for people to display symptoms of depression alongside insomnia. However, studies have been unable to determine which is the chicken and the egg and whether lack of sleep is caused by depression or whether depression is caused by lack of sleep.

The amino acid L-tryptophan that you will start using in Step 4 has serotonin-increasing antidepressant effects which may be sufficient to alleviate mild depression; however, if you are fairly certain that you have genuine depression independently from your insomnia you can find advice and treatment options on my website www. balancingbrainchemistry.co.uk and forthcoming book on sleeping brain chemistry for depression and bipolar syndrome (due for publication late 2014, see www.balancing brainchemistry.co.uk or my websites for details/publication dates).

The frontal parts of the brain, the parts involved in rational, cognitive thinking, become less functional without sleep and this impairs our ability to make rational judgements, leading to poor decision-making; this part of the brain also helps control impulsive behaviour and when it's impaired we may become irritable and short-tempered. Complex planning abilities and our perception of time also become compromised.

Poor mental performance and irritability can have significant social consequences which can easily be underestimated.

Physical effects of lack of sleep

An increased risk of several serious disorders has been linked to sleep deprivation, including hypertension, increased stress hormone levels and irregular heartbeat. Sleep deprivation can downgrade the strength of our immune system making us prone to infections.

SLEEP AND TYPE II DIABETES AND WEIGHT GAIN

Sleep-deprivation may cause weight gain and contribute to Type II diabetes.

In recent years an increasing number of epidemiological studies have found a relationship between insufficient sleep and the risk of gaining weight and Type II diabetes.

It has been shown that just a single night of lack of sleep increases the level of the hormone *ghrelin* in the blood which increases our appetite and drives us to eat more calories. It has also been shown that sleep deprivation results in people being less physically active and therefore they burn less calories. This dual effect of eating more calories and using less can obviously contribute to weight gain and acquired diabetes.

You'll find more techniques on my websites to help you lose weight by controlling your appetite (see Contact Details and Getting the Free Recordings); if you are overweight and have signs of sleep debt you should include improving your sleep as part of your weight loss regime.

If you have any of the above physical or mental problems and also have the signs of sleep debt discussed elsewhere use the techniques in this book to improve your sleep and overall health.

SKIN AND AGEING

Have you noticed how both parents show signs of rapid ageing during the years they have newborn babies disturbing their sleep? During our sleep the body increases its production of human growth hormone (hGH) which is responsible for regenerating and repairing tissues. Lack of deep sleep reduces the body's production of hGH. There's actually a way to use

GABA to increase the production of hGH and give you not only a restful but also an especially regenerated night's sleep; see www.balancingbrainchemistry.co.uk for details.

MELATONIN AND CANCER

Reduced levels of melatonin usually go hand-in-hand with insomnia and lack of sleep; as previously discussed decreased levels of melatonin are associated with a significant increase in your risk of developing cancer.

Take naps and siestas – they're good for you apart from when they kill you!

As already mentioned you would ideally avoid taking naps during the day so that at the end of the day you experience a greater pressure to sleep. An exception to this when you positively should take a nap and breaks the rule is when being too sleepy or actually falling asleep could cause dangerous accidents, for example when driving. If you are going to take a nap you will need to set an alarm to wake you up after a maximum of 45 minutes.

Taking short naps during the day is good for mental performance and appears to reduce mortality from all causes making you live longer, except after big fatty meals when taking a nap may kill you (Anthony and Anthony 1999; Rosekind *et al.* 1995).

A large study on the effect of napping and health was published in 2007 and showed that people who napped for half an hour at least three times a week had a 37 per cent lower risk of dying from heart attacks or other health problems compared to people who do not nap (Naska *et al.* 2007). Many years ago however I learned of research from 1964 (which I cannot find the reference to now) that sleeping after a big meal high in animal fats could trigger a heart attack upon waking. The theory is that, while lying still after a fatty meal, large fat droplets can accumulate within the lymph vessels in the abdomen and chest (the thoracic duct), then upon waking and moving all this fat is suddenly mobilised into the blood circulation and can precipitate a fatal heart attack within seconds after waking. All you have to do to avoid the possibility of this unfortunate demise is go for a walk or keep moving after a big fatty meal.

So it turns out that naps during the day are actually very good for you, improving not only your mental performance but your physical health and life expectancy as well. The exception to this is taking a nap after a big fatty meal like, for example, a Sunday roast or big dinner, where the effect may be to increase your risk of dying from a heart attack. The healthy thing to do after eating a big fatty meal is go for a walk or do anything that keeps you awake and moving around at least a little. Of course the really healthy thing to do is not eat the big fatty meals in the first place.

Research into the health consequences of napping is ongoing. A 2012 study suggests that frequent napping during the day in the elderly may significantly *increase* cognitive decline and the development of dementia (Ficca *et al.* 2010). If more definitive information emerges I'll post it on my websites, but for the time being a single short nap during the day appears to do more good than harm as long as it's not after a fatty meal.

Step 3: Mental exercises and recordings
Finding the positive source of your negative tension

1. You can lie down as you would to do a relaxation or sit for this exercise; you can do it away from your bed or lying in bed just before you fall asleep.

2. Now focus on and feel any tension you are holding. You may notice whereabouts in the body you feel it or it may simply be an emotional feeling. Just let

yourself experience it without reacting to it and ask yourself, what is the emotion in this tension?

3. Then ask yourself, why do I feel like this? and whatever the answer ask yourself why does this matter to me or what does that make me feel?

4. Keep asking yourself over and over again why does this matter to me, why does this bother me? until the answer you get has *positive qualities* and gives you *positive feelings*, when you will see it is something good you wish for or want as opposed to the original feeling, which was something unpleasant you don't want.

5. Now you must check, does this feeling come from a positive and healthy attitude or place in me, and is it truly what I (myself) want as opposed to something someone else in my life wants, or what someone else wants me to feel.

6. Once you have found the positive attribute at the core of the original stress and tension you felt observe the original feeling once more and you may notice that it has changed in some positive way, perhaps you feel differently about it.

Not only does this exercise help alleviate stressful feelings and therefore helps you to relax but it also and more importantly identifies the positive quality in you, the positive values in in your core self and what matters to you. Clarifying what matters to you can help you take the right steps in your life to achieving your goals, feeling fulfilled and less stressed.

7. If you do this exercise lying in bed as you fall asleep, imagine that you can programme your subconscious mind to work throughout the night like a computer doing an enormous calculation or search in the

background while you sleep. As you fall asleep ask yourself, what steps can I take in the coming days and weeks to fulfil and experience more of the positive values and beliefs that are important to me? All you do is ask the question and allow it to be passed over to your subconscious as you fall asleep. And you may be pleasantly surprised to find your subconscious mind can process problems for you as you sleep and that you notice helpful ideas coming into your conscious mind about the steps you can take that will move you closer to fulfilling your core goals.

8. You can take this a step further and ask yourself what do I really want to do? What is the one or maybe two things that I really want to achieve? You need to think about real-world things and be specific and clear. It's actually recommended to write down what you want; psychological studies have shown that people are more likely to achieve what they want when they write it down.

9. Now that you've clarified what's important to you ask your subconscious mind the question as you are falling asleep: what is the first practical and achievable step I can take to move me closer to achieving my important goals? The practical step may be a small thing like arranging an appointment, or maybe a big thing. Let your subconscious search through all your memory banks of accumulated knowledge and wisdom and work out the first and next step you need to take.

This technique can help you to let go of worrying about problems which may be keeping you awake, and instead allow yourself to fall asleep trusting that your subconscious will continue to help you solve the problem, tap into helpful areas of your mind and dream up solutions while you sleep.

You can use the above technique for big picture stuff or small goals and even before achieving better sleep.

Sleep recording 3
In this recording you will rehearse feeling relaxed and sleepy as you goes through the steps from your living room to your bedroom to stop your system producing stress responses at this critical time.

Summary of Step 3
In this step you start pre-loading the necessary supplements to help tackle your insomnia in the next step; you also learn about sleep and health. With the recording and mental exercises you will rehearse the ritual of going to bed without triggering a stress response that would otherwise wake you up and learn how to clarify and give up having to think about your daily worries, passing them over to the wisdom of your subconscious to come up with creative solutions while you sleep. The goal is that rather than daily worries keeping you awake your mind will be keen to go to sleep to solve your problems.

Putting Everything Together
Starting to Cure Your Insomnia

Your goals in Step 4

1. Start the bedroom timing and behavioural techniques to reprogramme your subconscious brain.

2. Start performing bright light therapy in the morning and strictly apply virtual darkness for 3–4 hours before it is time to go to bed. This will create a strong swing in your sleep–wake physiology.

3. Start taking the sleep-inducing supplements trystophan, theanine and GABA.

4. Perform a mental exercise to practise feeling sleepy.

5. The recording includes a mental exercise to diminish and eradicate feelings and beliefs that you are stuck with insomnia and to see its grip on you breaking up and letting go.

All the steps up to now have been important, but they were in a way only preparing you to do the better sleep treatment proper. This starts now by introducing some of the most powerful techniques to curing insomnia. In this step you will apply a multi-pronged approach to change both your physiology and your psychology.

You will affect your *biological clock* with bright light and darkness therapies. Adding the bright light therapy and darkness techniques to the B-12 and lithium you have pre-loaded for the past week will intensify the activity of your biological clock to send stronger signals to your body to wake up and go to sleep at the right times.

The combination of the tryptophan and light/darkness techniques will both increase the amount of the sleep hormone *melatonin* you produce and speed up how quickly you produce it, intensifying your desire to sleep.

The tryptophan, theanine and GABA supplements raise your levels of the *neurotransmitters* serotonin and GABA which calm the brain and are important for good sleep.

You will change your *subconscious association* with your bed (bedroom) with proven sleep timing techniques. These techniques should also make you very tired at the end of the day.

You will also practise useful new psychological exercises that will teach you how to induce feelings of sleepiness.

To really pile the pressure on to overcome your insomnia and kick-start better sleeping see if you can also be very physically active this week. Ideally you want to literally physically exhaust yourself, though even if you can't do this the other techniques will still work. Just make sure you're not physically *inactive*.

Lastly you will use the new recording, which will continue the parasympathetic relaxation training to eliminate elevated cortisol and the stress responses that maintain the alert *wake system* in your brain preventing your body from yielding to the *sleep system*. This new recording adds a powerful new subconscious exercise to diminish and eradicate feelings and beliefs that you are stuck with insomnia and to see its grip on you breaking up and letting go.

You can begin Step 4 as soon as you have:

- blocked out light from your bedroom

- got some blue blocking glasses for the evening

- got a bright blue light therapy device

- taken the B-12, lithium, magnesium, zinc and B complex for a week

- learned either the long slow breathing or the Buteyko breathing technique, whichever one feels the most relaxing for you

- practised the exercise where you imagine yourself feeling sleepy

- listened to better sleep recording 3 for a week.

Step 4: Supplements
Add:

- GABA: recommended dosage is 500 mg all the way up to 6000 mg, with 2000–3000 mg being an average starting dose. Can be taken with or without meals, to help you sleep take an hour or two before your bedtime. If anxiety and persistent thoughts are your problem take the higher dose of GABA.

- L-theanine 100–200 mg. Can be taken with or without meals, to help you sleep take an hour or two before your bedtime.

- L-tryptophan: dose 1000–1500 mg about 30 minutes before going to bed on *an empty stomach at least 2½ hours after dinner.*

Start the bright light therapy

Within an hour of waking up, either lying in bed or sitting eating breakfast, position a bright blue light therapy device within your visual field. Ideally position the light in the top half of your visual field, that is, above your central site line (imagine standing outside and looking at the horizon – that is your central site line and everything above it is blue sky). Positioning the blue light in this area optimises bright light therapy effectiveness by concentrating the light on the lower half of the retina where the maximum number of ipRG cells are located. Don't worry if it's inconvenient to place a light in this area, anywhere will do, just be consistent and do the same thing each day. Use a tape measure to position the device within 61 cm (24 inches) from your eyes and cut a piece of string to quickly measure the same distance every day.

The length of time you need to treat yourself will vary from person to person and with the strength of the device. The Philips Golite Blu will need at least 10 minutes and perhaps up to 20 minutes at full power. The much cheaper Syrcadian Blue SAD light therapy device would need longer, say 20–30 minutes. (See www.the-sleep-solution.com for the latest information and reviews of different bright light devices.) Remember the closer you position the device the shorter the treatment time needed, however you must follow the manufacturer's guidelines about the closest safe distance to use without causing eyestrain.

Working out the dose of BLT you need is simply done through trial and error; what you're looking for is an energised feeling within a few hours of the treatment. The feeling may only last an hour or so but it should be quite noticeable. Adjust the dose of your BLT to the minimum you need to produce this effect; you now know you are giving yourself a dose of BLT sufficient to influence your physiology. As a starting point try 15 minutes with the Philips device and 25 minutes with the Syrcadian Blue device.

For maximum effectiveness take your sublingual B-12 during your BLT treatment.

Reprogramming the subconscious with sleep and bedroom timing techniques

The sleep/bed timing techniques reprogramme the association your brain makes between your bed, insomnia and sleeping and its conditioned responses. At the moment when you think about going to bed you probably think about *insomnia* rather than sleeping well and that has to be changed. Have you ever had the experience of feeling sleepy or even falling asleep on the sofa but then as you get ready for bed, brush your teeth and go into the bedroom you wake up and then lie in bed with insomnia? Our subconscious mind has the ability to send signals via our nervous and hormonal systems automatically without even consciously being aware that it's doing this. Designed primarily to protect us from danger this automatic stress signalling system sometimes does not work well for us. Our subconscious mind is designed to learn and make simple associations; if you've lain in your bed many nights feeling stressed, worried, even angry about having insomnia your subconscious will automatically have learned to associate your bed and bedroom as stressful places. For the primitive subconscious stress equals danger and to keep you safe in threatening or dangerous places the subconscious initiates a stress fight-or-flight response which changes your internal physiology. Powerful life-preserving systems become active to keep you aroused, awake and prevent you being asleep. The negative mental association your subconscious has with your bedroom has the power to literally cancel all the physiological changes that were occurring in your body to begin a good night's sleep.

It's important to understand that the subconscious learns these associations and exerts its power over your sleep physiology automatically and it is *outside our conscious control*; in other words you can't just consciously think the problem away, or tell yourself to stop doing it. Fortunately behavioural psychology has discovered that the subconscious can learn the new associations and forget old ones. The subconscious makes new associations through repetition, all you have to do is repeatedly practise the new behaviour and your subconscious will automatically make and learn new associations. The sleep and bedroom timing techniques that you will begin in this step will remove unwanted programmes running in your subconscious that automatically control your physiology and stop you getting the sleep you desire.

Many people (sometimes called control freaks) feel uncomfortable with this notion and do not want to accept that there is a part of them that does things automatically, beyond the reach of their conscious control. A couple of examples of conditioned responses might help you accept that it is so: if I asked you to put your hand on an electrode and then repeatedly threw a switch in front of you which gave you a painful electric shock half a second later it wouldn't take long before you developed a *conditioned response* and moved your hand off the electrode as soon as I went near the switch. Your brain will learn this conditioned response automatically without you having to think about it, regardless of your beliefs. Even if I then showed you that I had disconnected the electrode from the electricity your brain would automatically yank your hands off the electrode when I threw the switch. Over time however you could unlearn the association between the electrode and the shock. You could produce a similar effect with blinking. If you repeatedly had water flicked in your eyes as someone raised their hand you would quite quickly develop a conditioned response and find it very difficult to not blink when they raised their hand, even as you just watch them dry their hands with a towel.

The cool thing is that the subconscious continues to learn and, with deliberate focused repetition of new experiences, we can imprint new associations and conditioned responses on it. You can think of your current sleep-conditioned responses as if they were programs in a computer and with the techniques in this section what you are going to do is overwrite the programmes that aren't working for you so that in the future your subconscious will associate going to bed with falling asleep and sleeping well.

Imagine how the subconscious programming of a really good sleeper works; as they are getting ready for bed, brushing their teeth, going into the bedroom, getting into the bed, their subconscious is doing the opposite to yours: it's switching *off* stress responses and *activating* sleep physiology. If you really apply all the techniques in this programme and work on training your mind you can gradually programme your subconscious to make it work like that in you too.

The sleep and bedroom timing rules

Every one of these rules plays an important function so do them all. They work on the subconscious parts of the brain that you cannot change simply by thinking or wanting to change; all you have to do is change your behaviour and your subconscious will automatically learn new conditioned responses. The effectiveness of these techniques has been developed over many years and tried and tested on thousands of people at Harvard and Massachusetts medical schools. The CBT programme included in what you're doing has been shown to help 90 per cent of patients reduce or eliminate their sleeping medication and 90 per cent of users report improvements. In this book you will use this tried and tested method and improve upon it with additional techniques.

1. SET YOUR ALARM AND GET UP HALF AN HOUR EARLIER THAN YOUR USUAL WAKING UP TIME.

This is going to be tough in the beginning if you've not had enough sleep but it's actually one of the most powerful things you can do to influence your sleepiness later on in the day. This extra half an hour in the morning will give you plenty of time to perform the bright light therapy, which you can do lying in bed as long as you're able to keep your eyes open!

If waking up early makes you feel tired don't worry because you can catch up sleeping the next night.

2. STICK TO YOUR SET WAKING UP TIME AND BLT SESSION EVEN AT WEEKENDS.

This is important to maintain the timing of your biological clock.

3. DON'T GO TO BED UNTIL YOU:

a. *feel genuinely sleepy.* Learn to recognise the subtle clues in your body that tell you your body wants to sleep *and*

b. *reach your threshold time for going to bed.* Your threshold time for going to bed is easy to work out: from the time you are going to get up count backwards the average number of hours you sleep (which you work out from your sleep diary) and that is your time for going to bed. So, for example, if you can wake up at 7:00 and you sleep an average of five hours a night your special time for going to bed is 2 a.m. You will be able to go to bed earlier in the future, as soon as you are sleeping better, but for now just stick to this rule, even if initially it means that you have to stay up very late indeed.

Insomnia can sometimes be quite an intractable problem and need strong medicine to get things going; natural therapies that successfully change your physiology and psychology without drugs often require a considerable input of effort, at least in the beginning. I encourage you to embrace a few days and nights of hardship to get the ball rolling.

4. START IMPOSING VIRTUAL DARKNESS ON YOUR EYES AT LEAST 3–4 HOURS BEFORE YOUR THRESHOLD SLEEP TIME.

5. DO NOT SPEND MORE THAN ABOUT 20 MINUTES LYING IN BED AWAKE TRYING TO FALL ASLEEP.

If you can't fall asleep within 20 minutes *get up and go to another room*. This may be a tough practice to do but it has been proven to produce results, even if it means you don't spend a lot of time in bed in the beginning you must still do it. It's important that you don't lie in bed clock watching, so just guess the time and estimate what feels like about 20 minutes. Also *within 20 minutes of waking up get out of bed*, after you wake up do not lie in bed watching TV, making phone calls, reading, etc.

One more point is that if you go to bed and don't feel sleepy any more just get up straight away, you don't have to wait 20 minutes before you get up.

6. DON'T TAKE NAPS DURING THE DAY THAT LAST MORE THAN 45 MINUTES, AND DON'T TAKE NAPS AFTER 2 P.M.

Ideally you wouldn't take any naps at all during the day to build up the maximum pressure to sleep later on; however, you can use short naps – even just ten minutes can improve energy and alertness.

Starting the sleep and bedroom timing techniques can be tough in the beginning and you will have to do some things that will probably feel uncomfortable. Just stick with it and remember why you're doing it: you have a subconscious part of your brain which learns really simplistic conditioned responses through repeated behaviour.

*Explanation and tips about the sleep
and bedroom timing techniques*

Making yourself wake up half an hour earlier, not taking long naps and not going to bed until you have passed your threshold bedtime *and* feel sleepy makes the day long, and this will build up the maximum sleep pressure. The more exercise, even just ten minutes walking, you can add to this the better. You goal is to make yourself tired and sleepy.

Many people with insomnia gives themselves permission to lie in at the weekends in an attempt to catch up on their sleep debt. The problem with doing this is it starts to change the timing of your biological clock, rolling it forward by two days and then making it harder to fall asleep on Sunday night. You then start a new week with another bad night's sleep and stressed about your condition. So until you become a master sleeper in several months' time you have to wake up and do your bright light therapy at the same time, even at the weekends. Occasionally, of course, you may have a late night on a Friday or Saturday, but you still have to stick to getting up early; all that will happen is you will be genuinely exhausted that day and actually probably sleep quite well the following night.

In the future, once your insomnia is cured, you may be able to allow yourself to sleep in at the weekends without it leading to insomnia by setting your alarm to your usual wake-up time, after which you could allow yourself to nap (if the BLT hasn't woken you up). Even though you sleep late in the morning the BLT session will still maintain the timing of your biological clock. This is an option for the future when you're cured and a good sleeper; for the next couple of months, however, get out of bed at the same time seven days a week, allowing yourself to take a short nap but not more than 45 minutes before 2 pm in the afternoon.

As you're going to be having to get up earlier than feels comfortable, including at the weekends, a good tip is to get an alarm clock that you like and gets the job done. I've noticed recently it's become commonplace for electric alarm clocks to have blue backlit displays, but blue light reduces and switches off melatonin production so it is a big mistake for manufacturers to use this colour. The only acceptable colour for any light source in the bedroom is red.

The combination of waking up half an hour earlier, sticking to that time at the weekends and not being allowed to go to bed until your threshold time, is the tough technique of the successful CBT insomnia curing programme. Many people find the staying up late an extremely unpleasant experience, even compared to what they normally do which is lie in bed tossing and turning stressing about insomnia. Actually it's a good thing, and the worse it feels the stronger and quicker the behavioural modifications will change your subconscious association, so embrace the feelings as a good thing like a good strong medicine that tastes horrible.

The other thing people often find very unpleasant is the exhaustion these adjustments can create in the first few days, and again this is a desirable thing, increasing the pressure on your system to fall asleep. If you feel exhausted during the day embrace this as a good effect of the treatment which will later on help you to sleep.

People with insomnia often go to bed early, hoping that maybe this night they'll fall asleep and have a good night; for example your sleep diary may show that you are only sleeping four hours a night but you may be spending eight hours a night in bed. This means that you are only sleeping 50 per cent of the time you spend in bed and this teaches your subconscious to make unhealthy associations between your bed and sleep. To reprogramme your subconscious you have to eliminate all the time you spend lying in bed *not* sleeping, even if that means staying up late in the beginning. For example, if you have to get up at 7 a.m. and your sleep diary tells you you're only averaging 4½ hours of sleep per night then your sleep threshold time is 2:30 a.m. and you literally have to stay up until that time! Initially this may sound too late but, if you think about it, what's the point in lying in bed when you are not sleeping? Try and be active in the evening rather than being a couch potato, some of the time switch off the TV and do some housework and prepare tomorrow's lunch, etc.

The purpose of the 20-minute rule is to change your subconscious associations with your bed and bedroom. We have to stop your subconscious brain associating your bed and bedroom with anything other than sleep. You're not allowed to lie in bed and wake in an insomniac state or doing other things such as reading, watching TV or using a laptop. *Basically only use your bed for sleep and sex.*

You will quickly learn to tell when it's time to get up and change rooms because you're not going to fall asleep quickly. You may feel tempted to stay in bed and hold out for the chance you'll fall asleep but don't; studies have shown that you will actually get more sleep on average by getting up and going to another room despite the feeling that it will disturb you and wake you up. In the other room you can read, listen to relaxing music, meditate and practise some of the mental exercises in this book until you feel sleepy again and return to your bedroom. What you must not do are things that are fun and reward you for staying awake, such as watching good TV or getting the housework done; you must not start anything that you need to finish and cannot just stop and walk away from, so you wouldn't want to start baking a cake or watching a thriller, for example. Reading and repeating the sleep exercises in this book are ideal activities.

You may feel bored, unhappy and want to do more engaging things, but it's actually part of changing the subconscious mind to avoid such rewarding things, even if it's unpleasant. The best thing you can do to speed up the onset of sleepy feelings is another session of one of the exercises or recordings from in this book. *You have to stay in the other room for at least 30 minutes* and *until you actually feel sleepy.*

The first goal of curing insomnia is just to *start* getting some better quality and more predictable sleep, even if it's only for a few hours; you will then be able to build from this small start and train your brain how to sleep better. Remember your body has automatic built-in sleeping systems that are trying to fix your problem every night. Your body wants to sleep and with the right treatment this natural process will start to work again. Once your mind senses signs of progress it begins to reduce the stress about sleeping that used to make falling asleep even harder, setting off a positive reinforcing feedback loop.

In the beginning some people find they have to get up and change rooms several times and may not get much sleep on the first night, however that should change on subsequent nights. Don't get disheartened and give up; as I said this part of the programme can be tough and temporarily make you feel *worse* before it makes you better. Because initially you may feel more exhausted you may choose to schedule the first few days of the programme away from important meetings, perhaps starting on vacation days. Remember that even though our conscious mind believes it is in charge and you cannot be simply programmed like a robot to change your associations there is another more primitive part of your brain that actually can be programmed by simple behavioural techniques. These techniques have been tried and tested on thousands of people and proven to be effective at kick-starting better sleeping.

You will probably start to experience better sleep quite quickly with the sleep and bed timing techniques but it's essential not to give them up straight away even if you think you are cured. Think long term and maintain the training to make sure you do not relapse and that in the future you become a sleep master.

Step 4: Mental exercise and recordings
Exercise to rehearse inducing sleepy feelings
Read these instructions through once before trying this exercise.

This exercise should be done just before you reach your threshold going to bed time and can be repeated if you wake up and had to change rooms.

1. Sit comfortably with your eyes relaxed and more or less closed.

2. Now think of a place where you remember you always slept really well like a log; if you don't have a place in mind, imagine such a place that will also work; otherwise just skip this step. Imagine looking at that place in front of you.

3. Now imagine there are people around you, perhaps friends, it's late in the day and they are yawning infectiously.

4. As you imagine the above scenes you feel yourself relaxing and your system cooling down internally.

5. Allow your mind to answer the following questions:

   ○ If falling asleep had a colour what colour would it be? Allow your mind to accept whatever colour comes to you.

   ○ If falling asleep had shape and texture what shape would it be, and what texture or material would be made from?

   ○ If falling asleep had a position or a place or a direction how would that be? Is it inside you and if so where in your body? Is it outside you and if so where is it around you and how does it move to you? Your answer could be something like this: falling asleep is like a soft black sphere in front of you which starts out small and then grows larger eventually enveloping you. Just accept whatever comes to you, however strange it may be.

6. Now put it all together: see the place where you sleep the best, it's late in the day and you are surrounded by people yawning and checking out for the night, imagine your system cooling down and intensify the qualities of falling asleep and sleeping. You don't have to force yourself to feel sleepy or fall asleep, just continue your imaginings and let it happen to you. For an extra nudge you can imagine all your waking thinking processes and thoughts being connected to a dimmer switch which slowly and gradually dims down and fades out your awake thoughts.

7. Continue this exercise until it makes your eyelids and head feel heavy and you feel the exercise is giving you the urge to yawn.

Sleep recording 4

Recording 4 includes a very powerful mental exercise to diminish and eradicate your feelings and beliefs that you are stuck with insomnia.

Summary of Step 4

In the previous three steps of this programme you had a lot to learn and get ready. From now on the learning gets much easier; there's nothing more to study. In this step you begin to put many techniques together to tackle your insomnia: you will apply rigorous bedroom timing and behavioural techniques to reprogramme your subconscious association between sleep and your bedroom; you will perform bright light therapy in the mornings which, coupled with the appropriate remedies, will influence your biological clock and improve your sleep; you will also apply virtual and total darkness at the other end of the day to maximise natural healthy melatonin production. Many people find doing the behavioural techniques makes them feel angry and unhappy initially but you've already suffered a lot with your sleep problem and invested a lot to get to this point in the treatment so stick with the proven behavioural sleep scheduling techniques and you can expect to notice the treatment changing your internal sleep physiology and psychology quickly.

You will also perform mental exercises to practise feeling sleepy, which will enhance your sensitivity to this natural process, and perform other exercises to dispel self-fulfilling beliefs that your insomnia is incurable.

Coming off Sleeping Pills, Building the Number of Hours You Sleep, Advanced Relaxation and Emotional Release Techniques

Your goals in Step 5

1. Learn how to build on the progress you've already made and gradually increase the number of hours you sleep a night to ensure you continue progressing.

2. Learn how to come off sleeping pills.

3. Perform advanced relaxation and emotional release techniques.

4. In the sleep recording you repeat and consolidate the previous exercises.

Building up your sleeping time

In this step you continue applying all the same bedroom scheduling rules. Once you are able to fall asleep quickly when you get into bed and sleep throughout the night, without having to get up and go to another room because you can't sleep, you can increase the amount of time you are allowed to spend in bed but it's important to *only make small adjustments*:

- If you have had insomnia for more than two years you are only allowed to add 15 minutes to your bedtime per night per week for the first two months, then 20 minutes per night per week thereafter.

- If you have had insomnia for less than 18 months you can increase by 20 minutes for the first month, then 30 minutes thereafter, but only increase if you are sleeping throughout the night.

- If you have had insomnia for less than a year you could try increasing by 30 minutes in the first month, but if you don't immediately achieve sleeping through the night 100 per cent revert to your starting position and then only allow yourself to add 15 minutes for the first month then perhaps 20, 30 and so on.

Golden rules

- Only increase time in bed when you are sleeping throughout the night without having to get up and change rooms.

- Increase by small increments only and observe if you continue to fill up the increased time with increased sleep.

- If you don't fill up all the extra time with sleep revert back to the previous schedule that was working for you for a week and progress in small increments. So if you try and increase 30 minutes and find it is too much, step back for at least a week and then when you're ready try 15 minutes.

You can add the extra minutes at the beginning or the end of the night although I recommend adding the extra time at the beginning of the night and sticking to the same wake-up time and bright light therapy session to fix the timing of your 24-hour biological clock.

The weekly increases mentioned above may not sound like much, and if you progress rapidly in your ability to sleep this 15 minutes per week rule may feel like it's holding you back rather than helping you. However, it's important to maintain a regular rhythm in your 24-hour sleep physiology and making larger changes can easily upset your sleep again.

Sleeping pills inhibit deep sleep, dreaming (REM) sleep and may kill you

Reasons not to use sleeping pills:

- Sleeping pills work by suppressing brain activity; the problem with this is that during deep sleep and REM sleep the brain actually becomes very active and sleeping pills therefore suppress deep sleep and REM sleep. Sleeping pills increase light stage two sleep only. Because sleeping pills inhibit the deep sleep phase you can still have a sleep debt the next day and feel tired rather than refreshed.

- One can quickly develop a tolerance to sleeping pills so that the dosage that previously worked is no longer as effective and you need to take a higher dose.

- Most sleeping pills create physical and psychological dependency which can make them difficult to give up.

- Last but by no means least *sleeping pills are associated with an increased mortality risk.*

Well-done studies have shown that taking even just a few doses of sleeping pills per month is associated with a significant increase in your risk of dying (Kripke *et al.* 2012; see also www.darksidedsleepingpills.com). As little as 18 sleeping pills per year is associated with a three and a half-fold increased risk of dying within the next 2½ years. People taking more than 132 sleeping pills per year had a 35 per cent increase in cancer (see Figure 3.3).

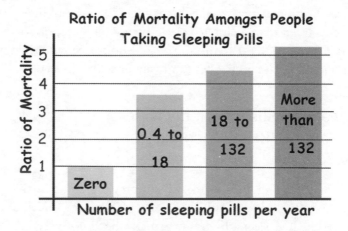

Figure 3.3: Mortality rate associated with taking sleeping pills

It should be understood, however, that the study did not prove that sleeping pills *caused* the increase in mortality; it only observed that people who took sleeping pills (also) had increased mortality rates. The fact that the more sleeping pills taken the higher the risk of dying does, however, make it look like it is the sleeping pills causing harm. More research is warranted to investigate this potentially very serious finding. For more information on this subject see the e-book *The Dark Side of Sleeping Pills* available free online (www. darksidedsleepingpills.com).

The bottom line with sleeping pills is that they only symptomatically assist you to manage insomnia, at best; they do not actually treat the condition nor help you in any way to a long-term cure. In fact they create a tendency which makes obtaining that long-term cure slower to achieve and taking them may damage your health.

The combined psychological and physical therapies in this book change the underlying problems, like lowering your evening cortisol and stress responses, eliminating light 'pollution', thereby increasing natural melatonin levels, and reprogramming subconscious associations with sleep. Together these therapies permanently change your natural sleep system.

How to come off sleeping pills

Unfortunately sleeping pills, particularly sleeping pills of the benzodiazepine family, can cause withdrawal dependency in some people so that they find they get rebound insomnia when they come off the drugs. If you are currently taking sleeping pills of the benzodiazepine type you may want to discuss with your doctor switching to a non-benzodiazepine hypnotic (those whose names start with the letter Z) because they have been found to cause less severe withdrawal problems.

Typically you can expect it to take 8–10 weeks to give up using sleeping pills. In my practice I regularly help people come off antidepressant and anti-anxiety medication and substitute natural safe remedies in their place; the typical reduction rate I recommend is 10 per cent a week or sometimes making reductions in 20 per cent steps every two weeks. It can be difficult to make small reductions like 10 per cent when you just have one pill; the fiddly but practical solution to this is to wrap the pill in strong paper and then crush it using the base of a bottle or a hammer. Then pour the crushed pill onto another piece of paper and arrange the crushed particles into a thin line (like making a line of cocaine if you're familiar with that from the movies) with a knife. Make the lines of even thickness then, using the knife, separate and push off the paper about one-tenth of the line and swallow what's left. Now you might think that the next week you just take away two-tenths but that's not what you want to do, because mathematically it means that each week you're making an increasing percentage reduction; you want to reduce medication by 10 per cent of what you're currently taking not 10 per cent of what you originally took at the start. It only takes an extra minute but what you have to do is form your usual line and take away 10 per cent of it, then draw the remaining line out back to the same length as the original line and take away one-tenth of this new thin line. If you're not mathematically orientated you'll just have to trust me on the maths here – do it this way and you'll maintain an even and consistent reduction; do it the wrong way and you'll start to make big and uncomfortable reductions. If you have the choice choose capsules rather than tablets, as you can just open the capsule and work with the powder. After seven weeks following this procedure you will have roughly halved the original dose and for simplicity you can now just remove 50 per cent of the line. You now have two choices: you can carry on at this half dose and start taking days off, say one day in every three you go to bed drug-free, then every two days you take a day off. If you continue to sleep well you progress so you only take this half dose every few days. You could also take melatonin on the days you don't take a sleeping pill. The other option is to continue taking an ever-diminishing daily dose; from the seventh week you draw the crumbled pill out into a line, remove 50 per cent with your first cut and draw the line out again to full length, take away one-tenth of that and continue as before.

You may find yourself having to juggle two things; as you start to sleep better you will probably want to increase the amount of time you are allowed to spend in bed using the 15-minute rule, but if you take yourself off sleeping pills at the same time you may find you're not able to progress your allowed time in bed. If at any time you stop sleeping well throughout the night take a step backwards and return to the previous higher dose of sleeping pills that was working and you may have to give up some of the minutes you added to your threshold sleeping time for a week or so until you're sleeping well through the night again.

I've met people who were taking sleeping pills and still not getting much sleep who decided that they wanted to just go cold turkey and give up the sleeping pills completely at the start of Step 4. If you want to do this I strongly recommend that you start taking melatonin as an alternative sleeping aid at the same time. You can't take melatonin indefinitely, so after six months or so with good sleep you could if you want to try slowly weaning yourself off the melatonin.

Why I don't recommend sleeping herbs

Herbal tablets and teas to assist sleeping have become very popular but I do not recommend them. They probably have a lot fewer side-effects compared to pharmaceutical medicines, however they are essentially doing the same thing and that is tranquillising your system rather than using light and dark to naturally reset your biological clock, prevent light pollution from blocking melatonin production, developing your relaxation response skills to stop your system over-producing cortisol at the wrong time of day and retraining your subconscious programming. It's even possible that some sleep-inducing herbs produce the same unwanted effect of increasing light sleep and inhibiting deep sleep. Perhaps there's a case for herbs as a very short-term stepping stone to help you transition off sleeping pills but I fear that you may end up with the same dependency and eventually want the stronger drugs. Despite my reservations you will find the page on herbs for sleeping on my website (www.the-sleep-solution.com).

Step 5: Mental exercises and recordings

You can use either one of these exercises, or both if you have the time. You need to allow yourself 20–30 minutes for each exercise.

Advanced relaxation and emotional release technique

Lie on your back as you do for your normal daily relaxation training but rather than going through your body and relaxing each part step-by-step perform the following exercise.

You can either use your mind to scan through your body and feel the area that feels the most tense or uncomfortable and then dwell on that tense and uncomfortable area and ask yourself, if this tension in my body had an emotion or feeling what would that emotion or feeling be? Generally you're looking for something unpleasant, anger, sadness, etc. Once you have identified the emotion and acknowledged it by admitting to yourself a part of me feels angry or sad or whatever, if you know what the feeling is about acknowledge that, and then, whilst simultaneously honouring the feeling and your right to have it, apply all your relaxation training skills and relax that part of the body and then progress on to relax all the rest of your body whilst still acknowledging that you have been holding that feeling.

Alternatively, as you lie on your back deliberately remember the painful, stressful, annoying or traumatic experience, and whilst holding it in your mind and acknowledging to yourself that part of you is still affected by this experience perform the progressive muscle relaxation technique that you've been training to do using the recordings. There are many ways you can use this technique, for example you could do it on a small scale, just going over the past day's events, or recall the significant stressful events of past year or your entire life; you could work from today and go backwards through time or you could start at the beginning and work forwards, acknowledging the key stressful events as they come into your mind; alternatively you could go straight to one key stressful event.

If you can train your system to go into a relaxation response and not produce the stress response whilst at the same time remembering unpleasant and stressful experiences you can train your system to sever the ongoing stress-producing effects of those memories and experiences.

To enhance the effectiveness of this technique take 200 mg of theanine or 1000 mg of GABA 20 minutes before starting the exercise. Adding these remedies puts the brain into an even calmer and less anxious state, which strengthens the message to your subconscious that you no longer produce stress response *in response* to these stressful memories.

N.B. This is a daily mental exercise and not a replacement for your daily parasympathetic relaxation response training.

Sleep recording 5
Recording 5 contains elements from previous recordings and exercises to consolidate and reinforce the subconscious changes you've made so far.

Summary of Step 5
Step 5 is about developing and progressing the gains you will have started in Step 4. You will gradually increase the number of hours you are allowed to spend in your bedroom without trying to rush things as the number of hours you spend sleeping increases.

During this step you will also finally give up sleeping pills if you haven't already done so. With the recordings and mental exercises you will develop and deepen your ability to relax and reinforce all the subconscious changes.

~ Step 6 ~

Consolidating and Perpetuating Your Gains

Your goals in Step 6

1. Continue practising the bedroom scheduling techniques from Step 4, adding more minutes until you're sleeping so well that you no longer have any signs of sleep debt during the day.

2. Continue weaning yourself off sleeping pills.

3. You can repeat any mental exercises that you have found useful to consolidate your progress.

4. Continue doing a daily parasympathetic relaxation response training to complete 100 days, either using my recorded instructions or following the written instructions available on my website (www.the-sleep-solution.com).

5. Sleep well for the rest of your life!

What to do if you have a bad night's sleep in the future

To reiterate, once you've overcome your insomnia and turned yourself into a good sleeper prevent insomnia from returning by responding quickly and aggressively to even a night or two of poor sleeping, thereby nipping it in the bud before it turns into a chronic problem. It's better to use 'overkill' for a week or so every once in a while rather than letting it slide into a chronic problem, when you would have to go through the whole insomnia cure programme again from the beginning. Incidentally that is something you can do, there is absolutely no physical or psychological reason why you couldn't do this programme more than once; every technique in this book can be repeated. It turns out that our subconscious programming is constantly learning and being updated anyway and just like in a computer you can reinstall the programme as many times as you want. But the simplest and most efficient thing to do is nip it in the bud as soon as it rears its head.

Let's say, for example, that you going through a period of extreme stress and that causes you to over-produce cortisol, keeping you awake in the evening. Immediately start practising daily relaxation response sessions, ideally as soon as you get home from work, to reset a relaxed condition in your body throughout the evening. Start supplementing extra nightly tryptophan, theanine, zinc, magnesium, B complex, B-12 and a bright light therapy session first thing in the morning if this is something you've stopped doing.

Step 6: Mental exercises and recordings

There are no specific mental exercises for Step 6; repeat any of the exercises you found helpful. You may not even need to practise them daily; perhaps two or three times a week over the next few weeks will continue and consolidate the benefits.

Sleep recording 6

The subconscious mental exercise in the final recording for this step is similar to the exercise you did in the first step in that it asks you to imagine yourself in the future and for evermore being a fantastic sleeper. In the first recording this may have felt like a distant, rather intangible, dream, but by now you should have made considerable progress and be sleeping much better and you ask your subconscious to see this continuing rather than imagine it's starting, as you did at the beginning.

Summary of Step 6

Step 6 is all about progressing and completing the sleep programme. You continue adding to the number of hours you are allowed to spend in your bedroom until you have reached sufficient powers to completely prevent any sensations of sleep debt during the day. To assist you in achieving this goal you can if you wish repeat any of the previous mental exercises or recordings that you feel address issues that were particularly problematic for your individual sleep problem. You continue weaning yourself off sleeping pills if necessary and it's very important to complete the 100 days of deep relaxation training.

PART 4

Restoring a Healthy Sleep Cycle

~ 4.1 ~

Sleep–Wake Cycles and Exposure to Light

With the protocols discussed in this section you can completely change the *timing* of your sleep–wake cycles. If you are a night owl and would like to become an early bird (or vice versa) you can. If you fall asleep too early in the evening to spend time with your family and then wake up at some ungodly hour all alone while everyone else is asleep you can change that. If you're a teenage night owl and want to be more mentally switched on for some morning exams you can do that also.

Controlling and maintaining healthy sleep cycles should be considered one of the cornerstones of successfully managing bipolar syndrome and people with this condition should use the techniques in this section. For more information on regulating sleep cycles for bipolar syndrome and depression see my website www.balancingbrainchemistry.co.uk.

As we saw in the introduction the timing of our biological clock is set by the timing of bright morning light and our biological clock determines the time of the release of cortisol, which gives us a surge of energy in the morning; and it is the absence of light in the evening that determines the timing of the release of melatonin that hits us with a wave of sleepiness at night. Since the industrial revolution many people receive inadequate bright light in the morning, due to working indoors, and too much artificial light in the evening to maintain healthy sleep cycles. Then there are people who have sleep cycles that are naturally too early or too late to fit in with the modern world and, finally, there are shift workers; this section is for all of these problems.

Today we get less bright light *and* less total darkness

Human light exposure has changed in industrialised societies. We evolved for thousands of years living mainly outdoors, exposed to natural daylight during the day and no artificial light at night, apart from a camp fire. We are designed to be exposed to these natural elements and, as we saw in the introduction, our biological clocks detect daylight and darkness and use these cues to run healthy sleep cycles.

In just a few hundred years since industrialisation people in developed countries have transitioned from working primarily outdoors regularly in bright light to working primarily indoors. This is not enough time for evolution to have changed and adapted our physiology.

Below are some figures illustrating the light levels in common settings. Light levels (or ambient brightness) are measured in *lux*:

- Very bright sunlight as on a ski slope may be greater than 20,000 lux; at this brightness and above most people will need to wear protective sunglasses to avoid snow blindness.

- A sunny day with a clear sky may be 10,000 lux.

- Daylight on a cloudy day may be 5000 lux.

- An hour before sunset may be 1000 lux.

- Fluorescent lighting in a brightly lit office may be 300–500 lux.

- A fashionable living room may be 50–100 lux.

- Streetlights or being 20 cm (8 inches) from a single candle may be 2–10 lux.

As you can see from the figures above the total amount of bright light we are exposed to today is a mere fraction of the light we used to be exposed to before the industrial revolution. Bright daylight with a cloudless sky will be about 10,000 lux, early morning light, especially under clouds, will still be 5000 lux but even a brightly lit office may be only 300–500 lux, as little as one-thirtieth of the light levels outdoors in sunshine. A typical office worker may rarely get exposed to bright daylight and this can prove inadequate to set our biological clock by, at least in some people.

The situation most likely also contributes to the development of depression by depriving us of the antidepressant effects of bright light.

Most discussions on health and exposure to light only focus on the *decline in the amount of bright light* we are exposed to and do not also consider the other big change, and that is that there has also been a significant decline in our exposure to proper darkness.

The development of electric lighting is obviously one of humankind's greatest achievements, however it is possible some people are supersensitive to the low levels of artificial evening light found in a modern home. Evidence from research has been contradictory on this subject but some studies (on people with bipolar) have shown as little as 200 lux (one-fiftieth of outdoor sunshine) can be enough to suppress melatonin production in some people (see my website www.balancingbrainchemistry.co.uk for more on this).

200 lux would be quite bright for a fashionable living room but common in brightly lit kitchens and bathrooms. Simply walking into a kitchen or bathroom in the evening

is sufficient in some supersensitive people to delay evening melatonin production and offset sleep cycles. As discussed another consequence of the decline in our exposure to proper darkness may be a rise in cancer rates, particularly breast cancer.

The temporary solution to this problem is wearing special amber-coloured glasses in the evenings; the more convenient and permanent solution is having alternative low blue light-emitting lighting in these areas.

In addition to some people being supersensitive to dim light it has also been proposed that some people may be too insensitive to *changes* in light intensity. They need to experience greater extremes or *contrast* in light intensity than the modern world gives them, that is their biological clock requires bright daylight in the day and pitch black at night. Indoor artificial light may be dimmer than the little bit of early morning daylight they experienced on their way to work but it may not be *different enough* to register with their biological clock, especially for people living in the far northern regions during the long winters.

Problematic Sleep Cycles

Night Owls, Early Birds
and Free Runners

Previously I said that the biological clock can keep quite good time all on its own, and whilst this is generally true it is possible but rare to have a biological clock that does *not* keep regular time. Even if the biological clock doesn't keep good time as long as we regularly get strong enough light signals via the eyes to reset the clock we can still be kept in sync with the outside world. In some blind people their biological clock does still receive signals from the eyes because the signals travel via different pathways to the optical nerves that give us sight. Other totally blind people, however, do not receive messages from the ipRG cells and if they also have a biological clock that does not keep to 24 hours their sleep–wake cycle progressively drifts out of sync each day; this is called a free-running sleep–wake cycle. This condition is common in blind people but considered extremely rare in sighted people. It has been my observation, however, that (sighted) people with bipolar syndrome quite commonly appear to have this non-24-hour-sleep cycle condition, but this may be a misdiagnosis.

Even when the internal body clock runs accurately at close to 24 hours you can still be out of sync with everyone else. There are some people who have a biological clock that works just fine, despite the way we work indoors without enough bright light in the day and too little darkness in the evenings with artificial light. Their problem is the *timing* of their biological clock is *out of sync with the modern world*. You'll find specific protocols for this problem below.

In some people their biological clock is shifted forwards or backwards, it keeps regular time but it's set later or earlier than most other people. Like a watch set to the wrong time their biological clock thinks it's in a different time zone and their sleep–wake cycles are out of sync with their work, shops, family and social circles.

So, for example, some people's 24-hour clock tells them to fall asleep early, at say 8 pm or even earlier, then to sleep eight hours and wake up at 4 am. This is called advanced sleep phase syndrome or *ASPS*. People with this early-bird sleep–wake cycle are perfectly evolved to be a livestock farmer like a shepherd or goat-herder in a pre-industrialised world. We'll look at ASPS in more detail later (see Figure 4.1).

Alternatively it's possible to have the opposite sleep cycle disorder, that is delayed sleep phase syndrome or *DSPS*. With this condition the internal clock is set late so you naturally want to go to sleep and wake up later than other people. Perhaps these night owls are naturally adapted for night-time hunting or night-watch protection.

Then there's a condition called non-24-hour or free-running sleep phase syndrome, whereby the internal clock does not run on a 24-hour cycle; it may be shorter, say 22 hours, but more commonly it is longer, say 25–26 hours. As a result the sleep–wake cycle progressively *rolls forward*, running later and later each day. Not only do people with this syndrome have an internal clock that runs too fast or too slow but they may be too insensitive to the light/darkness signals they experience day to day that should regularly reset their clocks.

There are also people whose biological clock would work just fine and would be in sync with the time zone they live in if they got enough bright light in the day and enough darkness in the evening; but their work schedule and lifestyle prevents them from ever seeing bright light/sunshine; alternatively they may do shift work and have irregular hours. It's impossible for me to suggest specific prescriptions for this problem because situations vary. Basically you should schedule regular bright light therapy at the beginning of your day and block out blue-light with amber sunglasses at the end of the day. You should be able to work out a way of improving your situation from the information in this chapter, but if this is your problem and you have depression or bipolar syndrome you may be better off changing your lifestyle and line of work.

Then there are other people whose biological clocks may be supersensitive to artificial light in the evening, delaying their sleep–wake cycle; these people need to set up virtual darkness as discussed in the Appendix 3. Alternatively, other people may be too insensitive to the little bit of dim morning light and contrast they get to properly set their biological clock; these people need to schedule bright light exposure in the morning and total or virtual darkness in the evening to establish greater contrast between the bright and dark phases of the day.

It has been suggested that the decline in exposure to bright light corresponds to the increase in the incidence of depression and the decline of exposure to total darkness may have contributed to the increase in the incidence of mania/bipolar. This makes intuitive sense, but whether or not this turns out to be proved, or even provable for that matter, remains to be seen. Interesting as that may be, the focus of this book is self-help treatment of sleep problems. In another book I will discuss how you can use bright light as an effective antidepressant and total darkness as an anti-mania/hypomania treatment (due for publication in late 2014, see www.balancingbrainchemistry.co.uk or my websites for details/publication dates).

All the sleep problems in this section are issues only in the *timing* of the sleep–wake cycle, the actual quality of sleep may be perfectly adequate. Difficulties with the *quality* of one's sleep or the ability to sleep at all (i.e. insomnia) are a different issue. Unfortunately the two types of problem are not mutually exclusive so you could have both a sleep phase disorder and poor sleep. See Part 2 on insomnia for help with this.

Circadian rhythm sleep disorders (CRSDs)

The circadian rhythm is the name given to your internal body clock. The 24-hour circadian rhythm regulates the timing of bodily functions like bowel movements, alertness, peak mental performance and the sleep–wake cycle, that is, when you naturally want to sleep and wake.

When the timing of your sleep–wake cycle is out of sync with the society around you it's called a circadian rhythm sleep disorder (CRSDs). CRSDs *result in a person being unable to go to sleep and wake up at times required for normal work, school and social needs.*

CRSDs can be caused by extrinsic or external factors such as jet lag or shift work. The focus of this chapter however is correcting *intrinsic or internally generated* CRSDs. These can take the three primary forms shown in Figure 4.1.

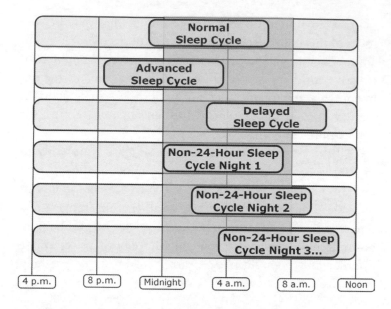

Figure 4.1: Sleep cycle disorders

- Normal sleep cycle (at the top): you fit in with normal social hours.

- Advanced sleep cycle: you fall asleep and wake too early.

- Delayed sleep cycle: you fall asleep too late and wake late.

- Non-24-hour sleep cycles don't run on a 24-hour cycle.

N.B. CRSDs are not a form of insomnia, there is no problem with falling asleep or with the quality of the sleep, it just all takes place at an awkward time.

The night owls: Delayed sleep phase disorder (DSPD)

People with delayed sleep phase disorder (DSPD) are the classic night owls; their biological clock runs on a regular 24-hour interval, it's just shifted so that their sleep–wake cycle runs later than fits in with regular school, work and social hours (i.e. they go to sleep late and wake up late).

DSPD is common and perfectly natural in teenagers, so much so that it has been argued by some educationalists and sleep scientists that schools should start later in the day and not do mentally demanding lessons such as mathematics in the beginning of the school day.

DSPD is common with depression and bipolar syndrome; using the bright light and darkness treatments discussed in this chapter not only helps sleep disorders but can also *directly* treat depression and bipolar syndrome. So using these techniques may be doubly beneficial.

As long as someone with DSPD can sleep in late and doesn't have to wake up before they have slept an adequate amount of time this condition presents no health problems from sleep deprivation. Sometimes labelled as lazy because of their tardiness in the morning, people with DSPD often find their brain becomes most alert, creative and productive about the same time other people are winding down and going to bed. The negative consequences of DSPD are the challenges it presents fitting in with the rest of the world. People with DSPD may have feelings of resentment toward authority because of being forced to get out of bed and work in a sleep-deprived state. Common consequences include performing poorly in morning examinations/meetings and sleep deprivation from waking up before they have had enough sleep, leading to poor immunity and ill health in general.

If you have DSPD you could try to get a job that involves doing late shifts, or use the treatment protocols below to alter the timing of your sleep–wake cycle to a time that suits you.

In brief, the basis of the treatment is to first pre-load the body with vitamin B-12 and low-dose lithium for several days, prevent bright light, especially blue light, entering your eyes in the evening and do intensive bright light treatments in the morning upon, or even before, rising. See 'Putting it all together' (page 214) for specific instructions.

Sleep and teenagers

An interesting field study (*ScienceDaily* 2010) demonstrated the power of virtual darkness by investigating the *negative* consequences of a lack exposure to bright blue light in the morning. Each morning teens wore amber-coloured glasses which block blue light and put them into virtual darkness. It was found that when blue wavelength light was blocked from entering the eyes in the *morning* their melatonin onset became progressively delayed by about six minutes each day the teens were exposed to virtual darkness. This adds up to a 30-minute delay in sleep onset after just five days, or potentially three hours in a month. This negative result cleverly demonstrated the powerful effects of controlling exposure to blue light with virtual darkness. Of course, we want to bring sleep on earlier, not delay it, so we will impose virtual darkness in the evening not the morning.

Too much artificial light in the evening and lack of bright light in the morning could have huge implications for student performance. Sleep onset typically occurs about two hours after melatonin onset. To improve studying and exam performance students should use bright blue light therapy in the morning and virtual darkness in the evening. Teens should follow the light/dark schedule for DSPD.

The early birds: Advanced sleep phase disorder (ASPD)

This disorder is characterised by falling asleep early in the evening and early morning waking. It is often seen in the elderly. For a person with ASPD the natural time to go to sleep may be as early as six o'clock in the evening, which may be totally impractical with work and family commitments. This can cause lack of sleep and health problems when a person is unable to go to bed early enough in the evening to get enough hours sleep before their usual early morning wake-up time. The sleep deprivation that people with ASPD typically suffer may cause sleepiness during the afternoon.

People with ASPD have a sleep–wake cycle that is perfectly tuned to livestock farming in a pre-industrialised world. The traditional shepherd or goat herder lived outdoors, fell asleep shortly after sunset and awoke very early with their flock at the first glimmer of light before the sun even appeared above the horizon. For a farmer there are plenty things to do at four o'clock in the morning and by midday or early afternoon they may have finished a full day's work so eating dinner at 5 p.m. and falling asleep by 7 p.m. would be normal.

For the 9–5 office worker, on the other hand, waking every day at 4 a.m. can be a miserable and lonely experience and falling asleep at 6–7 p.m. is too early for family and social life.

It's interesting to note that before the widespread adoption of electric lighting from the late 1900s onwards ASPD would not have even been considered a problem medical syndrome at all. There was little to do in the evenings after dark without cheap electricity powering up lights, televisions and now computers.

People with ASPD could consider getting early shift work that suits their nature, like being a postman. Alternatively, by using the techniques described in this chapter you can adjust your sleep cycle to whatever time you want.

Basically you need to pre-load the body with low-dose lithium for several days to facilitate the transition, use black-out blinds in your bedroom to completely prevent any dawn light signals reaching your eyes and use bright lights in the afternoon or early evening to offset melatonin production. See 'Putting it all together' (page 214) for details.

The free runners: Non-24-hour sleep–wake disorder

This used to be called free-running sleep phase syndrome. In non-24-hour sleep–wake disorder the internal clock runs longer or shorter than 24 hours *and* is not being reset by outside light signals. Typically the person's internal clock will run on a 25 or 26-hour cycle, rarely it can be even longer; in one documented case the person would stay awake for 48 hours then sleep for 24 hours on a regular scheduled basis, they were perfectly healthy when allowed to follow their own unusual sleep–wake cycle.

The consequence of having an internal clock that runs an hour or two longer than 24 hours is that the sleep–wake cycle gets pushed back each day and continually rolls forward. If the person yields to their natural sleep cycle they would end up going to sleep later and later, eventually going to sleep during the day at very unorthodox times. If they try to maintain orthodox sleeping times, periodically every few weeks their sleep–wake cycle ends up in sync with normal working hours and every few weeks they are completely out of sync, awake during what is their night, causing a very tired, groggy, late-night appearance and condition. It is basically akin to taking a sleeping pill during the day then going about your business.

Obviously, left untreated, free-running sleep phase syndrome will disrupt a person's ability to maintain both work and social engagements. In extreme cases people have resorted to home-schooling/working to cope with this condition.

As already mentioned non-24-hour sleep–wake disorder is very rare in sighted people; however it may occur in more than 50 per cent of people with total blindness. The nerve pathways from the ipRG cells in the eye, which convey signals to the biological clock, travel along a different route to the nerve pathways that give us sight and in some blind people the pathways still work, telling them when it's daytime. However, sometimes the nerve pathways are not functional and the person's biological clock never receives light signals telling them when it day or night. Gradually their biological clock moves out of sync with the outside world.

In sighted people with non-24-hour sleep–wake disorder, however, the problem may be not that their biological clock is unable to receive signals from outside light and reset itself but rather that their reset mechanism is relatively *insensitive* and only works when exposed to *strong* signals from intensely bright light and genuine darkness. Perhaps for these people today's indoor living and working just does not provide strong enough signals to reset the internal clock. Their day may involve exposure to early morning (not particularly bright) light for just a few minutes on the commute to work, followed by all day working indoors, then hours of electric light, TV and computer screens in the evening, there may even be 10 lux in their bedroom. Pre-industrial people would have regularly experienced days that ranged from almost zero lux on moonless nights to several hours of 10,000 lux outdoors. Even if the biological clock was only reset every few days it would not free run.

Although it appears that the contrast between the maximum brightness and darkness during the day may be significant in resetting our biological clock in some people, it is not understood how important contrast is, and even if it has a significant impact at all; it's just a theory born out of observation. What is clear from the research is that *bright light exposure plays a central role in resetting our biological clock*, and this is something we can easily control.

To treat non-24-hour sleep–wake disorder in sighted people I would strongly recommend you include both bright light *and* total darkness to intensify and exaggerate the contrast of the light/darkness signals and not just add bright light.

I believe some people may appear to have non-24-hour sleep–wake disorder, because they keep sleeping later and later but, rather than being essentially blind to light signals and unable to have their biological clock reset, they are instead supersensitive to even a low level of electric light in the evening and this light keeps offsetting their melatonin production and pushing their sleep cycles back.

I would be very interested to hear if any blind people with this condition have tried to treat it using the Valkee bright light therapy device that shines bright light into the brain through the bones of the skull via the ear canals. See the section on choosing a light box on www.the-sleep-solution. com for more information.

The treatment for non-24-hour sleep–wake disorder is basically the same as DSPD, the only difference being that when you start to reset your sleep–wake cycle to normal social hours you don't know where your cycle is currently running. Your 24-hour clock could be running many hours apart from normal social hours and starting a treatment could result in a dramatic shift in your sleep cycles. It's not going to be terrible, just a bit disorientating. I've been told when you publish a cookbook you should test every recipe three times, so I deliberately made my sleep cycle delayed and brought it back to normal three times to test these methods. On the last test I shifted my sleep–wake cycle 11 hours in five days and in the more uncomfortable east to west travel direction. The adjustment was remarkably easy and *completely free of jet lag symptoms*, my internal clock simply jumped to a markedly different time within about 30 hours of administering the light/darkness phase of the treatment protocol. See 'Putting It All Together' (page 214) for specific treatment details.

As mentioned sleep cycle disorders only affect the *timing* of your sleep, they do not affect the *quality or quantity* of your sleep. In fact it's been observed that people with non-24-hour sleep–wake disorder typically have better quality sleep than the average person when they allow themselves to sleep at their own rhythm.

Sleep rhythm disorders are almost always going to have *physiological* and not psychological cause, unlike insomnia which may significantly involve psychological issues.

≈ 4.3 ≈

How to Adjust Your Sleep Cycle

The sleep cycle disorder medicine chest

Next we'll look at the remedies and procedures you need to correct and move your sleep–wake cycle to wherever you want. To retrain your sleep–wake cycle you'll need the following:

- a bright light device

- a very low-dose lithium supplement

- a very high-dose sublingual B-12 supplement

- the early birds need to set up totally light-tight darkness in their bedrooms and a pair of amber-protective glasses if they make early morning trips to the bathroom

- the night owls need a virtual darkness set up for the evenings.

Supplements for sleep cycle disorders

There are two sleep remedies, lithium and B-12, that can help us to shift the timing of our sleep–wake cycles.

Lithium

As discussed in Chapter 1.2, lithium directly affects the enzymes used by our biological clock and supplementing lithium can improve the functioning of our biological clock to control sleep cycles.

B-12 Methylcobalamin

Also as discussed in Chapter 1.2, B-12 increases the effectiveness of bright light therapy and speeds up the rate at which melatonin is released in the night and stops being released in the morning.

Without lithium and B-12 supplements some people find BLT will keep them awake, with these supplements BLT helps you sleep.

To reap the benefits it is essential to choose the right type of B-12 supplements and use it properly (see the B-12 section in Appendix 2).

Bright light treatment and darkness for sleep cycle disorders

BLT has a central role in treating CRSD; it sets the timing of the biological clock.

There are many cheap and ineffective bright light therapy devices on sale; and the technology keeps changing, so for up-to-date information on how to choose an effective bright light device see my website (www.the-sleep-solution.com).

For instructions on how to perform a bright light therapy treatment see 'How to Perform a Bright Light Treatment' in Appendix 1.

The importance of using darkness for problems with sleep cycles

It is not clear precisely how important darkness is in resetting the biological clock. It appears that bright dawn light sets the *timing* of the biological clock to its 24-hour position and the onset of darkness informs the biological clock how *long* the day is so that our body knows what season it is and when to release melatonin at the end of the day. In some animals determining the season tells them the right time of year to make babies.

In totally blind people and when people live in 24-hour darkness the suprachiasmatic nucleus coordinates the timed release of melatonin, however under normal circumstances, as long as light continues to enter the eyes, melatonin production is delayed. In other words, sufficient bright light in the evening overrides the suprachiasmatic nucleus and curtails melatonin production.

Previously the decline in bright light in our modern world has been highlighted as a cause for increasing rates of depression (Kirpke *et al.* 1994). There is now mounting evidence that adequate darkness is also very important to our health and that too much artificial light after sunset disturbs our sleep and increases our risk of cancer (Hansen 2001; Reiter *et al.* 2007; Stevens 2006).

By removing *all* light from your bedroom you prevent the morning sun being able to signal to your biological clock when the day has started. You can now choose the time you want to receive that first light signal and adjust the timing of your sleep–wake cycle.

By making your bedroom totally dark you are also creating more extreme *contrast* between the intensity of the light and dark phases of your day. This would help people whose systems may be too insensitive to light/dark signals for the modern world, with electric lights in the evening and little/no bright outdoor light during their day.

Making your bedroom totally dark also increases melatonin production which helps insomnia, reduces cancer risk and protects the brain from ageing.

Making a room completely light tight takes a little work; for advice on how to do this see 'How to Set Up Virtual and Total Darkness' in Appendix 3.

Virtual darkness for sleep cycle disorders

As already discussed, research has found that only blue/cyan light stimulates the ipRG cells in our eyes that send signals to the biological clock. Therefore if we eliminate all blue/cyan light in the evening the ipRG cells are no longer simulated, for them all the light has gone out and your biological clock 'thinks' we are in real darkness. This signals to the pineal gland that it's time to start making melatonin and within a couple of hours melatonin levels rise. In the virtual darkness environment the other light sensitive cells in the eyes – the ones we use to see the world with – still work so we can carry on with our evening activities without artificial light signals offsetting our sleep–wake cycle.

Creating virtual darkness for several hours before you want to fall asleep is sufficient to adjust your sleep–wake cycle. If you want to get the most benefit (anti-cancer/ageing) from your natural melatonin start the virtual darkness every day several hours before you go to sleep so that *the total time you spend in virtual darkness and asleep in real darkness adds up to 12 hours.*

Remember you must not interrupt the virtual darkness even briefly. It's no good, for example, blocking blue light for several hours before bed then exposing yourself to regular light, to brush your teeth or remove makeup. Even a fairly brief exposure to bright light can switch off melatonin production for several hours.

People with DSPD (i.e. late sleeper/risers) want to bring *on* earlier and stronger melatonin production to go to sleep earlier. They should at least dim down evening lights and ideally set up virtual darkness. They must absolutely avoid *all* bright light exposure in the evening for several hours before they want to sleep.

There is evidence that at least some people with bipolar syndrome are supersensitive to even low levels of light, switching off their melatonin production, so using virtual darkness in the evening can be especially important/useful for living with bipolar syndrome.

If you have ASPD on the other hand, you want to *delay* melatonin production and stay awake later in the evenings. So you should *expose* yourself to bright light in the late afternoon and early evening to offset your sleep cycle; you can use bright lights potentially up to two hours before you want to sleep, though personal experimentation is advised.

Putting it all together: How to adjust sleep cycle disorder

With the use of supplements, BLT and the specific use of darkness/low-blue light the body takes only a couple of days to adjust the timing of your sleep–wake cycle. With the protocols described in this text you can move your sleep–wake cycles with minimum discomfort and a very brief transition period. You can switch from a life long of being a night owl to an early bird or vice versa. You may be amazed to find you experience your normal day, just at a different time!

Setting up the total darkness can be quite challenging, it is probably only strictly necessary if you are an early bird with ASPS or you have bipolar syndrome. For night owls with DSPS the most important objective is imposing total darkness and excluding disturbing light pollution in the evening and applying BLT early in the morning.

Despite the effort it is worthwhile setting up a totally dark bedroom and virtual darkness or at least diminishing evening light because of the health-promoting benefits, including cancer-fighting properties, of increased natural melatonin. See Step 1 for more information on evening light pollution and cancer risk.

With a few simple changes to curtains and taping over bright light sources on clock radios, etc. you should be able to significantly dim down the light levels in your sleeping area, and you can also wear an eye mask. This may be dark enough for night owls with DSPS, but remember the more you avoid bright/blue light for several hours before sleeping and the darker your bedroom the more melatonin you will make, which has additional health benefits.

The problem with adjusting sleep cycles

Responses to BLT can vary from one individual to another so personal experimentation is required. However personal experimentation that involves disrupting your sleep cycles may be a potentially hazardous process. By disturbing your sleep cycle you could end up sleep deprived, drowsy and mess up an important meeting or, worse still, have an accident. Supposedly after 17 hours without sleep our cognitive performance declines in an equivalent way to the decline you would get with a blood alcohol level of 0.05 per cent which is the legal drink drive limit in the UK. I remember the case in the late 1990s of a man who fell asleep whilst driving; he survived but his vehicle derailed a train killing several people. The subsequent court case concluded he had had too little sleep for several days prior to the accident and he went to jail for manslaughter.

When adjusting your sleep–wake cycles it's very easy to inadvertently change one end of the cycle, either waking up or falling asleep, and not the other end. So you might start waking up at the crack of dawn by using bright morning light, but still be going to bed late because you have not dimmed down bright evening lights. Alternatively you may stay awake later in the evening by using bright evening light but still wake up very early in the morning because you still allow early morning sunlight to enter your bedroom.

The solution

The therapeutic trick I've discovered to make moving your sleep–wake cycle a smooth, insomnia and jet lag symptom-free transition is to pre-load *specific supplements into your system for at least five days and ideally a week before commencing the BLT.*

As far as controlling bright light and darkness goes, gather together and set up everything you going to need, the bright light device, the low-blue lights, yellow glasses if you are going to use them, blackout blinds for the bedroom windows, etc., and start changing both ends of your sleep–wake cycle simultaneously, but don't start this until you've prepared your system using supplements as outlined below.

As already discussed, supplementing B-12 intensifies the pineal gland's melatonin response to both bright light and darkness. Pre-loading vitamin B-12 sets us up for this effect to kick in as soon as we start the bright light and darkness treatments. In addition to supplementing B-12 you should also pre-load a low dose of lithium from Lithinase. Lithium *directly* regulates the 24-hour body clock and supplementing it smoothes out and speeds up the transition as you change the timing of your sleep–wake cycle.

Using this combination of supplements prior to starting the BLT reliably prevents the BLT from potentially wreaking havoc on your sleep–wake cycles.

People with bipolar syndrome (type I or II) should also pre-load EPA rich fish oil if they are not already on it – along with extra lithium – to counteract the risk of BLT inducing mania/hypomania.

If your work or situation absolutely could not withstand the possibility of a little insomnia or drowsiness I would recommend clearing your schedule of important concerns for the first two or three days you start to use BLT, just in case your sleep–wake cycle bounces around and you need to take a quick nap during the day.

Treatment for early birds: How to shift ASPS (early rising/early sleeping)

For ASPS you'll need:

- to create total darkness in your bedroom to completely prevent any dawn light penetrating

- to have blue-light blocking sunglasses or low-blue bug lights for nocturnal bathroom visits

- a reasonably powerful bright light device (say 2500 lux).

You don't need to be concerned about avoiding blue light in the evening and probably don't need a 10,000 lux white light box or high-end blue LED bright light device. With ASPS the supplements may not be strictly necessary but would still be helpful, especially the Lithinase. *Setting up the total darkness to completely prevent your eyes from receiving early morning light is, however, absolutely essential and not an option.* See 'How to Set Up Virtual and Total Darkness' in Appendix 3.

There are several ways get the bright evening light. You can buy one of the very expensive designer bright lamps often sold alongside SAD light boxes (for example the Kubo SAD lamp). Perhaps the best option is to buy a low-cost SAD light box costing about £35 ($50). Like the expensive designer lamps these cheap light boxes typically produce 2500 lux at usable distances from the lamp. This may not be bright enough to produce much of the antidepressant effect very bright lights can, but is sufficiently bright to offset melatonin production and manage ASPS. Any bright light will probably do, however, so to save money you could simply use 2–3 energy efficient 25–36 Watt light bulbs behind a thin white or bluish lampshade.

PROTOCOL TO TREAT ASPS

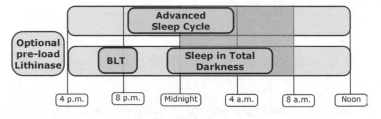

Figure 4.2: Therapeutic protocol for ASPS

The top line illustrates your current sleeping position and the bottom line how to use light and darkness and move your sleep time.

1. Set up total darkness in your bedroom *before* starting BLT.

2. If you get up in the night for bathroom breaks you will need to wear blue light-blocking glasses.

3. Optionally take two Lithinase capsules last thing at night for one week prior to starting BLT, it helps to regulate the sleep–wake cycle and will assist you through the transitional period while you experiment with how best to perform the BLT.

4. Begin with two hours of BLT at about 2500 lux (see manufacturer's guidelines) in the evening, stopping three hours before you would like to sleep. This is just a suggestion to begin with and you should experiment to get the effect you want. You should increase the intensity of the light to the point where it makes you feel quite awake; to increase the

intensity of the BLT sit closer to the bright lights or upgrade to a more powerful/blue light device. To perform the BLT all you have to do is have the bright light somewhere in your visual field while preparing food, eating or watching television.

5. Once you've achieved the results you want you can discontinue the Lithinase.

People with ASPS don't tend to have problems either falling asleep or waking up on time and therefore probably would not benefit from B-12 supplementation.

Treatment for night owls and free runners: How to shift DSPS (late rising/late sleeping) and non-24-hour sleep–wake disorder (free-running sleep–wake cycle)

For DSPS you'll need:

- to eliminate bright and blue light in the evening; ideally set up virtual darkness

- a high end, powerful SAD light box/device (see Appendix 1 for recommendations)

- all the supplements outlined below.

You don't need to be concerned about creating total darkness in your bedroom, just dimming down extraneous light will suffice.

You will need all three of the above components, nothing is optional.

BLT can easily take care of the earlier waking-up time you want to achieve, but you will need B-12, Lithinase and low blue light in the evening to make you fall asleep earlier.

Protocol for DSPS

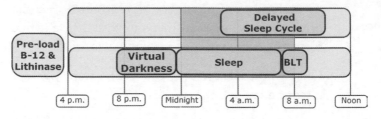

Figure 4.3: Therapeutic protocol for DSPS

The top line illustrates your current sleeping position and the bottom line how to use light and darkness and move your sleep time.

1. Make whatever changes you need to in order to avoid bright light especially blue light in the evening. The best and easiest option to live with is to create virtual darkness by using yellow low blue light in the evening especially in your kitchen and bathroom. Other options include installing dimmer switches and dimming down all your lights, your computer screens and TV, etc. in the evening. If you spend a lot of time on the computer in the evening it is worth investing in an amber-coloured computer screen cover.

2. For one week before starting BLT pre-load the following supplements:

   ◦ Hold 2000 mg sublingual B-12 lozenge under your tongue in the morning and in the evening.

   ◦ Take two Lithinase capsules with dinner.

3. After one week on the supplements commence the BLT. From now on you take your morning B-12 during the BLT and your evening B-12 several hours before the time you would like to sleep. If you forget and miss the time just take a catch a dose of B-12

when you've remembered. For a gentle start on the first day expose yourself to the BLT as soon as you wake up and then that night try anything and everything you can like herbal teas, meditation, melatonin supplements, etc., to have an early night.

4. On the second day and until your sleep cycle has moved to where you want it to be set your alarm for an hour before the time you want to wake up and do BLT when the alarm goes off. You do the BLT at this time even if you don't intend to get up straight away, and snooze for a while. Doing the BLT at this time may even mean you don't get a very long night's sleep, but it will help a quick transition. What you are doing is simulating a bright dawn, initiating the shutting off of melatonin production and resetting your biological clock. From now on you must *look out for the natural wave of tiredness* that rising melatonin levels brings on in the evening and *pack yourself off to bed when that feeling arrives.* You must do this even if it seems to be far too early compared to what you're used to. Do not override this sleepy feeling; if you override the feeling it may pass and you'll miss the opportunity it gives you to change your sleep cycle. This step may require a little discipline in the beginning, but it is part of the retraining of your sleep–wake cycle; if you feel like you're losing time in the evening, remember you will get it back in the morning.

If your sleep cycle does not move to the time you want it to after a couple of days of performing the BLT an hour before you want to wake up you have two options:

1. You could move the timing of the BLT treatment earlier, up to two hours before you want your body to naturally wake up.

2. You can try increasing the intensity of the BLT by increasing the length of the treatment or, for a stronger effect, shorten the distance you position the bright light device from your eyes.

Once your sleep cycle has moved to the time you want it to you could try doing the BLT at a more comfortable time after you have woken up, either whilst still lying in bed or soon after getting up. After a couple of weeks try stopping the lithium, taking half the dose for a few days, then every second day, for a few more days before finally stopping. Without the B-12, however, you may not get a rapid release of melatonin sending you to sleep in the evening. You can probably take both doses in one go from now on for convenience, but you'll have to experiment and see.

Some people don't like to take supplements long term and may want to wean themselves off the B-12. If that's the case for you, are you reading the right book?! Remember there are *no negative consequences* from taking high doses of B-12 long term and it may keep ageing homocysteine levels low.

Mental creativity and changing your sleep–wake cycle

Many people with a delayed sleep phase will say that their mind becomes the most switched on and productive very late in the day, even when some people are thinking of going to sleep. Unfortunately you may find your mental creativity does not immediately adjust and peak at a new earlier time in the day, so if you use your mind for creative work you may initially feel you don't have your usual sharp edge. Gradually your system changes, however, and within a week or two at the most you'll be able to do earlier in the day everything you used to do.

~ 4.4 ~

Jet Lag

Travelling east

Most people's biological clock finds this the worst direction to travel in, in terms of jet lag. When travelling east you effectively end up with DSPS at your destination. If you can organise it, when you first arrive avoid morning appointments and sleep in late according to local time.

Basically you want to prepare by doing progressively earlier morning BLT and virtual darkness in the evening. Below you'll find a full involved protocol and a simple version.

Protocol to speed up/prevent jet lag when travelling east

- Pre-load Lithinase/B-12 for a week before travelling (see DSPS protocol on page 220).

- Before you travel do a day of BLT in the morning and virtual darkness in the evening for every two time zones (two hours' time difference).

- On the first day of treatment set your alarm clock an hour earlier than usual and perform the BLT for 30–40 minutes. On the second day do the BLT two hours earlier, on the third day do the BLT three hours earlier, etc. Impose virtual darkness on yourself in the evening and try to advance your bedtime an hour earlier for every hour earlier you get up for the BLT.

This will not move your biological clock to exactly the same time as your destination, but it will move it about halfway, offset the jet lag and allow you to carry on your routine before you travel pretty much as normal.

For example, if you are travelling six time zones do the BLT/virtual darkness three days before you go, on the first day you do the BLT one hour earlier than your normal wake-up time and try to go to bed an hour earlier after one hour virtual darkness (this means you start the virtual darkness two hours before you normally go to sleep). On the second day do the BLT two hours before your normal wake-up time and try to go to bed two hours earlier after an hour of virtual darkness, etc. Even if you can't manage to go to bed earlier keep imposing the virtual darkness.

- You can even start the virtual darkness the night before your first BLT session.

- Optionally advance your meal times; eat your breakfast, lunch and dinner progressively earlier.

- Once you arrive at your destination avoid morning light before 10 a.m. for a day or two by sleeping with an eye mask on and wearing amber blue-blocking glasses; even just wearing sunglasses will help.

- Perform BLT mid-morning until you fully adjust to the local time.

This protocol will help a lot but you may still feel a bit out of sync; if you don't want any jet lag stay at home!

The simple version

- Take the supplements for several days, especially the Lithinase, you would benefit from the Lithinase even if you only take it when you arrive.

- Avoid bright light in the evenings; ideally wear amber sunglasses and do BLT as early as you can in the morning for a couple of days.

- Then, when you arrive, strongly impose the local time on your eyes by doing BLT when you get up in the morning (local time) and wear amber glasses in the evening from, say, 8 p.m. This will send strong signals to your biological clock and encourage a faster transition.

Melatonin for jet lag

You can use melatonin supplements for jet lag. The evidence is contradictory whether melatonin actually helps to entrain the biological clock or it just helps you sleep. Use it freely whenever you want to make yourself sleep during travelling. See Appendix 2 for recommended use.

Travelling west

Generally people have little or no difficulties with jet lag when travelling in this direction.

When travelling west you effectively end up with ASPS at your destination. If you can organise it when you first arrive avoid evening appointments and late nights.

Basically you want to prepare by doing progressively later evening BLT and virtual darkness in the morning when you wake up.

Protocol to speed up/prevent jet lag when travelling west

- Pre-load Lithinase for several days before travelling.

- Before you travel do a day of BLT in the early evening and impose virtual darkness in the morning for every three time zones (three hours' time difference) you travel.

- For the virtual darkness strictly block out all exposure to early morning light in your bedroom and as soon as you get up impose virtual darkness on yourself with amber (blue light-blocking) glasses. Wear the glasses for one hour for every three time zones you travel, starting with 1–2 hours on the first day and adding an hour every day.

- Do a 30-minute BLT session in the late afternoon or early evening and try staying up later each day

- Optionally delay your meal times; eat your breakfast, lunch and dinner progressively later.

- On the day of the flight wear amber blue light-blocking glasses or at least avoid all bright light and wear sunglasses until after 2 p.m.

- Once you arrive at your destination stay up until *local* bedtime.

- Now you perform BLT upon rising in the morning and wear amber glasses in the evening until you fully adjust to the local time.

This should be sufficient to ease your transition when travelling west.

The simple version

- Take the supplements for several days, especially the Lithinase, you would benefit from the Lithinase even if you only take it when you arrive.

- Avoid bright light in the mornings; ideally use amber glasses or at least sunglasses and do BLT in the evening for a couple of days.

- Then, when you arrive, strongly impose the local time on your eyes by doing BLT when you get up in the morning (local time) and wear amber glasses the evening from, say, 8 p.m. This will send strong signals to your biological clock and encourage a faster transition.

Appendices

Appendix 1
How to Perform a Bright Light Treatment (BLT)

For up-to-date advice on choosing a bright light device see my website (www.the-sleep-solution.com).

CAUTION: If you have bipolar syndrome don't use bright light therapy until you have good control over your mania/hypomania and have already started total darkness treatments. See the chapter Bright Light and Total Darkness Treatment in my book on depression and bipolar syndrome (due for publication in late 2014, see www.balancingbrainchemistry.co.uk or my websites for details/publication dates).

All modern bright light devices are designed to be ultraviolet (UV)-free and eye safe; there is no evidence that modern bright light devices cause eye damage. To be safe and avoid UV eye damage buy a properly made bright light device from a reputable supplier; only try and make your own if you understand the light spectrum and what UV is.

All you have to do to perform a BLT is have the bright light device positioned within your visual field, that is, behind, in front or to the side of whatever you're going to look at throughout the treatment, then stay looking in the same general area more or less continuously throughout the treatment. Reading, eating, watching TV or using a computer are obvious things you could do.

Doing BLT with basic white light box (the original light boxes)

If you are going to use one of the original type white light boxes you will need to spend more time performing the treatment than if you use one of the newer blue light devices.

To treat ASPS you may be able to get satisfactory results with a 2500 lux light box; these are quite bright but you can certainly watch TV and use a computer at the same time. To treat DSPS or get a significant antidepressant effect from bright light treatment, on the other hand, you will need a more powerful device, producing 10,000 lux. These very bright white light devices are so bright, however, it's like having car headlights shining in your eyes; you cannot comfortably watch TV or use a computer. You'll see sellers' websites depicting people using a light box whilst watching TV or using a computer, but don't be misled into thinking that you can use a 10,000 lux bright light device and do these things at the same time.

Using these old style white light devices made doing BLT a bit unpleasant and a bit of a hassle. Having one of these light boxes in your line of sight is so dazzling it makes viewing a computer or TV screen at the same time quite difficult.

I've found there are only three things you can do during BLT with one of these devices:

- First, you could do nothing else but just stare into space while listening to radio or music for example. You could do this for 30 minutes while still lying in bed.

- The second thing you can do is read printed material laid flat just in front of the light box. Kindles and other e-readers would also work.

- Third, you could put a meal in front of the light box and eat while you *look at your food*. Focusing on your food when you eat it, so-called conscious eating, is actually a technique that is proven to reduce overeating and help weight management.

Although they are usable, as outlined above, I always found white light boxes unpleasant to use. Despite this the benefits far outweighed the inconvenience and discomfort. Imagine being able to overcome your sleep problem and/or improve depression with a few supplements and half an hour in front of a bright light while reading or eating. If you don't already own one of these devices get one of the modern blue light devices.

Doing BLT with a new blue light LED

The new blue LED bright light devices are so efficient at stimulating the ipRG cells that they do not have to be anything like as bright as the original white light boxes and in my opinion have revolutionised bright light treatment, both for moving circadian sleep cycles and for treating depression. They can be positioned next to a computer monitor or laptop, just in front of you, between your eyes and a TV without being too dazzling and causing interference. Some of the devices, like the Philips Golite, allow you to change the brightness level so that it can be adjusted to suit your eyes.

Whatever unit you use it's essential to give yourself a *consistent dosage* of light each session. Without consistency you will not be able to establish your ideal dose and, worse still, you may accidently overdose, running the risk of disturbing your sleep or inducing a manic/hypomanic episode if you have bipolar.

There are three variables that change the strength of the treatment:

1. the *distance* between the device and your eyes

2. the *intensity setting* you select on the device – if that's an option

3. the *duration* of the session.

I suggest you fix and don't change the first two then experiment with the duration of the session only.

Of the three variables changing the distance between your eyes and the device makes the biggest and a somewhat unpredictable difference. This is because the intensity of light from a source decreases exponentially with increasing distance. What this means in practice is that if you change the distance between your eyes and the bright light device by more than 13 cm (5 inches) or so you *significantly* change the intensity of the treatment. For this reason always maintain a consistent distance between your eyes and the device and use the same distance each treatment session. Casually placing the device in front of you and then leaning forwards, backwards or from side to side, as you use the phone, for example, is too inconsistent and may cause you problems.

To achieve this all you need to do is work out a simple measurement using your arm and always set the device at exactly the same distance from your eyes. Use a tape measure to establish the range of distances recommended by the manufacturer, then with your shoulders squared off, use your arm and see where the device comes to on your wrist or hand. Choose a distance within the manufacturer's recommended range that falls nicely on something easy to use like your knuckles or the pad of your palm, then use this measurement to achieve daily consistency.

You don't need to fix your eyes still on one precise spot, all you need to do with your eyes is keep the bright light device somewhere in your visual field, so just keeping your head pointing in the same general direction will do. Focusing on reading material, a crossword, Sudoku, your breakfast, a computer or TV gives you something to do. I tried carrying my device around clocking up a couple of minutes brushing my teeth, buttering my toast, etc. but the results were just too inconsistent; so you do need to stay in one place. I'm sorry to labour this point so much but being inconsistent in the distance between your eyes and the device can significantly change the intensity of the treatment. A possible alternative approach may be provided by the latest 'wearable' bright light devices that allow you to move around.

If you're using an old-fashioned white light box you'll need to stay close enough to the light box to receive about 10,000 lux hitting your eyes for 30–40 minutes or 2500 lux for 2–3 hours. You'll need to know from the manufacturer how many centimetres/inches your eyes will have to be from the device to achieve these brightness intensities. It's impossible to calculate the exact brightness equivalents between the white light boxes and the newer blue LED bright light devices; you will see manufacturers suggesting their blue light device is equivalent to 10,000 or 5000 lux but this is a bit of a guess. They do, however, still come with a minimum and maximum recommended distance, and you can experiment from there.

If your device allows you to select different brightness levels choose a level that strikes a balance between being noticeable and unobtrusive. Obviously the brighter the setting the shorter the treatment needs to be.

Fixing the above two components leaves you to experiment with the only remaining variable: the length of the treatment.

The exact treatment time needed to achieve the results you want varies from person to person; so, as with all the other techniques described in this book, you'll have to experiment. As a starting guideline try somewhere between 15–45 minutes each session with a blue light device or a 10,000 lux white-light. At 2500 lux the treatment times may need to be 2–3 hours, so 2500-lux devices are not strong enough to be practical for treating DSPS; who has the time to sit in front of one of these things for 2–3 hours in the morning? They could work in the evening watching TV for people with ASPS but why not just buy a more powerful blue light device and you will be able to give yourself a much shorter treatment. As little as 15–30 minutes of bright blue light exposure could give you the boost you need to stay awake and change your ASPS.

With supplements I often recommend starting at the maximum dose to see how they make you feel and then scaling down, but with bright light I recommend starting with a middle dose for several days and adjusting from there to avoid insomnia; people with brains that can become manic/hypomanic should probably start with a low dose on the first day and build up; however, if you have already set up total darkness therapy as I recommend, you should be able to quickly antidote any problems with darkness and a few supplements.

Using a timer, increase or decrease the session time in 10-minute blocks, or 25 minutes if using 2500 lux. Personally I observed the effects of changing the treatment within 1–3 days, so I found it easy to adjust and establish my ideal dose. Some people respond more slowly, making it harder to determine the best dosage. What I would do in that case is keep a journal of the length of each treatment and your sleep patterns for a few weeks. From this journal you will be able to establish how many days it takes between changing the treatment time and it affecting your sleep. Once you have this number you know how many days to look back to see what you did and establish the length of treatment that works for you. Generally your body will be quite consistent in how long it takes to respond to changes in the dosage of BLT. This may all sound like a lot of work but you only have to do it once for years of benefit.

Position in your visual field

Because the ipRG cells are predominantly located in the lower part of the retina that receives light from above it is believed that light hitting the eyes from *above your line of sight* has a more powerful therapeutic effect. This makes sense, since this is where the blue sky is normally positioned within our visual field. I don't use this approach myself and the treatment still works, so this refinement is not essential; maybe if did add this I could reduce the treatment time.

Appendix 2
How to Choose and Use the Right Type of B-12 Supplements

Choosing the right type of B-12

Most B-12 supplements contain a cheap, synthetic form of B-12 called cyanocobalamin. This form of B-12 does not occur in natural foods, however it can be converted in the body into the active form of B-12 called methylcobalamin. The downside of cyanocobalamin is that it does not efficiently supplement the active ingredient we want, and in the process of conversion to methylcobalamin it depletes the body of valuable methyl groups that control inflammation in the body. Cyanocobalamin may be acceptable for short-term use to correct B-12 deficiency or for occasional use by vegans and vegetarians whose diets supply inadequate levels of B-12.

For long-term use, however, you must buy B-12 supplements containing *methylcobalamin only*. I once accidentally bought cyanocobalamin and found that it was still capable of influencing my melatonin production, but much less efficiently and I had to take four times as much to achieve a similar effect.

Properly using B-12

Vitamin B-12 is not well absorbed by the digestive system, with perhaps as much as 99 per cent of what is ingested passing right through the body unabsorbed. To efficiently get B-12 into the body we want to bypass the digestive tract. The most efficient way to do this is through injections directly into the bloodstream; alternative routes are directly through the skin or directly under the tongue. Skin patches are available at considerable expense, however, leaving sublingual administration as the best non-prescription, non-injection option. Sublingual B-12 supplements can be a very efficient way to get B-12 into the body, but only if it's a well-made product and you use it properly.

When choosing a sublingual format make sure you get a sublingual tablet that very quickly dissolves under the tongue. Many manufacturers sell B-12 lozenges that you suck like a boiled sweet, effectively swallowing the B-12 in the saliva it generates. Some of the B-12 will be absorbed under the tongue but most is swallowed and once in the intestines only 1 per cent is absorbed, so these lozenges are basically little better than swallowing a tablet. A true sublingual is quite different, it dissolves very quickly under the tongue, within say 90 seconds, and the B-12 is absorbed directly into the bloodstream through the blood vessels under the tongue. Some poorly designed sublingual pills do not dissolve quickly, and you need to crush the lozenge ideally between two spoons or in folded paper into powder/small crumbs that will dissolve quickly. You can crush the pill with your teeth and push the pieces under your tongue, but this often does not work well as the bits tend to stick to your teeth and you end up swallowing most of what's produced.

For a sublingual to work you need to hold the saliva containing the B-12 under your tongue for 2–3 minutes without swallowing, which is actually harder than you might think. With practice the technique becomes easy.

I recommend:

- *Source Naturals* methylcobalamin sublingual 1000 mcg

- *MRM* methylcobalamin 2000 mcg

- *Life Extension* methylcobalamin lozenges 1 or 5 mg

- *Jarrow* methylcobalamin 2000 mcg. (Generally a dose of 2000 mcg works best.)

The above products are too hard to be called proper sublingual supplements; however, if you crush the tablet with your teeth then hold the crumbs under your tongue you can make them work. The difficult part is that when you crumble the tablet you get a burst of flavour and experience an intense desire to swallow the excess saliva, but *you must train yourself to resist the urge to swallow and hold all the B-12 under your tongue*. You can swish the saliva under your tongue if you want. I know it may sound like I'm going a bit over the top with detailed instructions, but the B-12 has to be held under the tongue to be efficiently absorbed; remember 99 per cent of what you swallow is not absorbed by the intestines.

- Superior Source Microlingual methylcobalamin 1000 mcg.

This manufacturer has produced a true sublingual product that dissolves almost instantly. The small tablets are made from lactose, however, and are therefore not suitable for lactose-intolerant people. They also produce a higher 5000 mcg B-12 with 800 mcg folic acid and 2 mg B-6, which would be a simple effective daily supplement to keep homocysteine levels low as well as help our sleep cycles and mental health. Elevated homocysteine may be involved in promoting ageing of the brain.

You may need to experiment to establish the dosage of methylcobalamin you need to create the desired effect, but typical doses to affect melatonin production from the pineal gland are 2000–3000 mcg (2–3 mg).

Are high doses of B-12 safe?

Yes, very safe. B-12 is so non-toxic that it has not yet been possible to establish a toxic dose, even at ridiculously high doses no toxic effect has ever been observed. You could swallow an entire bottle of B-12 per day without toxic effects. This is great news because it allows us to use the high doses needed to affect melatonin production and lower homocysteine without any safety worries.

Appendix 3
How to Set Up Virtual and Total Darkness

Making your bedroom light tight
Windows

Making your bedroom completely light tight in a convenient and permanent way may take some time and you may not want to wait to do this before moving forward with the rest of the insomnia programme. So you could consider in the meantime setting up some temporary light-blocking measures: you could temporarily duct-tape thick black plastic sheeting or cardboard over your bedroom windows, roll up a blanket and put it across the bottom of the door and hang thick heavy cloth over the door on temporary picture hooks; you may need to hang a heavy curtain on both sides of the door if that's what it takes to block out all the light.

You probably won't want to live with these measures in the long run so look online for sources of blackout blinds for the windows. Be warned, however, that many people selling blackout blinds are actually just selling roller blinds made with light-proof material which only partially do the job. What happens is the fabric of the roller blind will never rest flush with the window frame and make a light tight seal, so what you will need to do to make these kind of cheaper blackout blinds completely light tight is install a strip of wood just like a picture frame in front of the roller blind so that the sides of the blinds run behind this picture frame setup and the light will find it impossible to turn the corners and come into the room. You can buy strips of wood shaped like a letter L that do the job perfectly. That takes care of the sides, now for the bottom and top; the bottom is easy, you install the L-shaped picture frame strip along the bottom with a hole drilled in the centre for the draw cord from the blind to run through, you simply pull up lying down by hand pulling the string out as you go and finally use a string to pull the blind snugly down the last few centimetres into the light tight frame. The top is a little more complicated, light will come up behind the back of the roller itself, bounce off the window frame and come into the room so you need to effectively box the roller in so that the light coming up behind it is caught inside the box.

You can buy ready-made off-the-shelf completely enclosed light tight blinds but obviously they're more expensive. You could buy blinds made with blackout material and then make them completely light tight yourself, it's actually quite easy. The general principle is light travels in straight lines and can only turn corners by reflecting off the surfaces it hits so paint the back (hidden) side of the picture frame with matte black paint or stick some black fabric like velvet to it and this will absorb the light rather than reflecting it. When making a photographic blackout darkroom the general rule is if you force the light to turn and bounce around three corners that is sufficient to stop it entering. A good tip for DIY products like this is to construct a temporary mock-up out of cardboard and tape to see how it will work and visualise the project in your mind. Once the project is finished a lick of paint and none of it will look out of place.

Doors

Blocking the light out around the door is actually quite easy. Use either flat or L-shaped (for recessed doors) strips of wood on the outside of the door frame (i.e. the opposite side to the way the door opens) essentially picture-framing the door.

That way the door opens freely but when shut it closes up against the extending picture frame and this forces light to bounce around the inside of the door frame and the picture frame to escape. To make it light tight make the inside of the picture frame black with either paint or velvet. Again you might want to try a mock-up using cardboard just to clarify what you need to do. Incidentally using black velvet on the inside of the light-blocking picture frames on the windows and doors turns these light-blocking systems into great draught excluders, increasing the insulation of your home.

For the bottom of the door frame simply attach a draught excluder to the base of the door.

When you've done the above jobs properly you should be able to stay in the room for a few minutes during the middle of the day, allowing your eyes to adjust to the darkness, and not be able to see any light coming in around the windows or the doors.

Also, as a quick start and for when travelling, get a well-fitting eyemask.

Internal light sources

You will also need to consider sources of light you have in the room such as clock radios, etc. If they give off exclusively a deep red light than they are acceptable, however other colours of light are not and will need to be replaced or covered up. As a quick temporary start you can tape black paper, cardboard, velvet or aluminium foil over all non-red sources of light in your bedroom. Be careful not to block the heat escaping vents on electrical equipment. No TVs, computers or tablet devices, including bright mobile phone screens, are allowed to be on in the bedroom.

Bedroom lighting

To get started you can change the light bulbs in your bedroom for very low powered dim bulbs or why not just straightaway buy some yellow bug light bulbs for your main bedroom light and bedside light. If you prefer to have a little background light in your bedroom you can get amber/red nightlights that plug into the wall socket or see if you can find one of the old red photographic darkroom lamps, which actually give off quite a pleasant romantic light.

Creating virtual darkness in your evening living area

To set up virtual darkness and induce earlier melatonin production you can do the following:

- get special yellow-coloured light bulbs that emit hardly any blue light

- wear amber-tinted blue-blocking glasses (see below) in the evening

- dim down your computer monitor and perhaps your TV if you have a LED backlit TV, as these emit a lot more blue. You can even buy amber-coloured low-blue screens that you fit over your computer monitor in the evening; they are available online.

Also, in general, dim down interior evening lighting, and all light bulbs you use in the evening must be completely screened by an amber/orange red shade. By completely screened I mean you must not be able to see the naked bulb directly with your eyes. Even the brief flashes of bright light you may experience by glancing directly at the naked bulb can offset your melatonin production.

In the living room dimming down lights is quite easy to do; the real problem arises when you go into the kitchen or the bathroom to brush your teeth. These areas tend to be brightly lit and you'll be entering them with your pupils wide open from your dimly lit living room. This will potentially expose the retina of your eyes to melatonin-blocking levels of light. There are two solutions to this: you can either install alternative low-blue lights in these areas; or wear amber-tinted sunglasses that filter out the blue part of the light spectrum. You may not always want yellow lights in your kitchen; my set up is to have the yellow bulbs in the main overhead light sockets and have alternative white lights on the counter top to provide white light in the day and mornings; a low-powered light box would be perfect for this.

The amber-coloured glasses must be large enough to prevent direct light coming in from around the sides and over the top, they also need to be a specific amber tint that block almost all wavelengths below 540 nm. See www.lowblue-lights.com and my site www.the-sleep-solution.com for more information.

The cheapest source of amber/orange coloured safety eyeglasses is Uvex S0360X Ultra-spec 2000 safety eyewear orange frame SCT-Orange available from Amazon for about $10. You will not win any fashion awards, to be honest they make you look a bit scary, but they get the job done and effectively block out the specific blue light frequencies that influence melatonin production, and are a great way to get started on increasing your melatonin production and overcoming insomnia, especially if you are on a budget. A word of warning: I have seen what appeared to be the cheap low blue safety glasses available from Amazon for about $10 being sold in the UK for £199!

Because increasing melatonin production has such powerful health-promoting effects you may want to set up more permanent and user-friendly ways of creating virtual darkness in your evenings with the use of yellow light bulbs in the bathroom and kitchen areas, etc.

You can also tell your optician that you want sunglasses to eliminate blue light; they will be able to make some blue-blocking glasses for you.

The yellow light bulbs are sometimes called bug lights, as they are reputed to repel insects. Search online for 'low blue lights' or 'yellow bug lights', they again are available from Amazon. If you install yellow bug lights in your bathroom and kitchen I would still recommend getting a pair of low blue-blocking glasses; you'll find them useful for occasional use.

I'm sorry, but brightly lit makeup mirrors are absolutely forbidden at night. It has been shown that even a relatively short burst of bright light shuts off melatonin production for several hours.

Studies have related poor sleep and an increase in breast cancer among women who remove their makeup last thing at night using brightly lit makeup mirrors (Blask 2009; Gooley *et al.* 2011; Wahaschaffe *et al.* 2013). It was proposed that the reduced antioxidant benefits of melatonin cause an increased cancer rate. However, it may also have been to do with the poor quality sleep compromising the immune system.

Tablets

For the same reason you must not use a tablet or computer screen for 3–4 hours without wearing low blue light protective glasses or covering the screen with low blue screen covers, available online. One study showed that two hours exposure to a backlit tablet device (tablet computers, iPads, etc.) prior to bedtime reduced overall melatonin production by 22 per cent (Wood *et al.* 2013). All you have to do to prevent this is use an amber-coloured screen cover or amber-coloured glasses.

Backlit LED TVs

The new backlit LED TVs give off significantly brighter and more blueish light than older TVs. Wearing amber glasses is the only real option for watching one of these TVs for three hours before you sleep.

Appendix 4
Choosing and Using the Right Melatonin Supplements

It's probably a good idea to keep a diary with some kind of rating scale (length of sleep, depth of sleep, quality of dreams, morning drowsiness on a scale of 1 to 10, etc.) to help you conduct your melatonin experiments.

The variables are:

1. the delivery system (instant or timed release)

2. the dosage

3. the timing, that is, how long before bed to take it

4. different brands can produce different effects.

First, do you need *time release, instant release, regular release or a mixture of these*?

- For difficulty with *staying asleep* and waking up use time release.

- For difficulty with *falling asleep* use instant release lozenges or regular release tablets. If you have both problems use a mixture of regular release and time release.

Second, what is the *best dose* for you?

For some people higher doses between 3–5 mg are best; for others, however, these doses can cause nightmares and lower doses, between 300 mcg–1 mg, produce the best results. Incidentally these very low doses are more comparable to the amount of melatonin naturally produced by our own pineal gland.

I recommend that the first time you buy melatonin to buy very small capsules (300 mcg) and experiment to find your preferred dose; try from 1 to 15 capsules (i.e. 0.3 mg to 4.5 mg). Once you've found the ideal dosage you could buy that size capsule in the future.

Third, if your problem is falling asleep experiment *with how long it takes before the melatonin makes you feel like sleeping*. Try taking it one, two, three or four hours before bedtime. For a while I found it useful to take a low dose (300 mcg) at the time of sunset or 7 p.m., whichever was the later.

Lastly, it's surprising how different the effects can be with different brands. I recommend trying a bunch of manufacturers and expect to give some bottles away unfinished because they don't suit you.

Appendix 5
Recommended Meditations

If you're resistant to the idea of meditation I encourage you to just temporarily suspend your scepticism, follow the instructions properly and see what happens.

Any calming, peaceful meditation may be helpful to sleep, but here are some particularly useful techniques. Meditation before sleep help to destress the body and mind and reduce cortisol levels. Meditation performed at the same time each night in the bedroom may also help to get you into your bedroom and away from your TV/computer.

Below are some meditations I found particularly helpful to encourage restful sleep.

Left nostril breathing
This yoga breathing technique can work wonders, try it.

Lie in bed on your left side, resting a thumb or finger on your right nostril to close it. Make your breathing *slower and deeper*, that is, engage in long, slow, deep breathing entirely through the left nostril. That's pretty much all there is to it, you could optionally add any relaxing, soothing, self-healing/blessing affirmation you want to at the same time. Expect to continue this meditation exercise for at least 20 to 30 minutes; keep going until you fall asleep. This technique is considered 'cooling' in Oriental medicine terms and so is particularly recommended when overheating and or menopausal hot flushes are causing sleep difficulties.

The six healing sounds

This is a Taoist meditation technique published by a Mantak Chia (available in DVD (recommended) or book format from www.universal-tao.com or online booksellers). This technique is based on the Oriental medicine idea that we store different emotional tensions in different body organs: anger in the liver and worry in the spleen, for example. Performing specific sound vibrations shakes free and discharges the accumulation of pent-up emotions from the organs. Use this meditation to destress last thing at night just before sleep. An important point which was not explained in earlier versions of the six healing sounds book is that you should continue to repeat each sound (in sets of three according to Taoist doctrine) until you *experience* a release and cooling effect with regard to the feeling you're working on. So, for example, a person with pent-up anger may need to do the liver sound (associated with anger) many times, say 27 or 30, and all the other sounds only three times to get the job done. Basically you keep going until you've cleared all the pent-up emotions from the day (or the whole of your life up to that point the first time you do it!). And go to sleep with a clean slate. It's an interesting and useful mental process and I cannot recommend it highly enough. To learn this technique I recommend purchasing the DVD or download version instructions rather than the book, available from www.the-sleep-solution.com; you can probably find samples of it on YouTube also.

Sub-vocally chanting om

Lie comfortably on your side and repeatedly, slowly chant 'om' on your outbreath. Do it quietly to start with, gradually reducing the volume until it's only barely audible, or even sub-audible. Similar to the left nostril breathing above, you should expect to have to continue this practice for at least 25 minutes, and perhaps much longer, until you fall asleep.

I'm sure you can find people chanting 'om' on YouTube to get you started.

Slow pranayama versus Buteyko

A small percentage of people find that when they do slow 'yoga' breathing, instead of making them feel calm it makes them feel agitated and panicky. If this happens to you the Buteyko method of breathing is usually the solution (see Part 3, Step 1). Most people find the Buteyko method produces the desired effect of calming the nervous system.

Breathing apps

Saagara have made a wonderful app called Universal Breathing for the iPad/iPhone and other formats that helps you do a guided slow breathing meditation; see Pranayama on their website (www.saagara.com). There's a free light version for you to try before you buy. Normally you do meditations sitting in an upright position with a perfectly straight spine, however you could use this app and do the slow breathing lying on your back, in your totally dark bedroom.

A kundalini yoga trick I was taught was to make a commitment to doing your chosen meditation for 40, 90 or 120 days continuously in a row, without missing a single day. If you miss a day you have to go back to the beginning and start counting from one again! It's a useful discipline trick; try it.

Glossary

ADENOSINE

A chemical that is a by-product of energy production that builds up continuously in our cells as we produce energy every hour we are awake, and is broken down as we sleep. In the brain adenosine acts like a tranquillising neurotransmitter gradually building up a strong pressure to sleep so that after 16–18 hours without sleeping adenosine makes it increasingly difficult for us to stay awake, requiring ever-increasing levels of cortisol and adrenaline to override it.

ADVANCED SLEEP PHASE DISORDER (ASPD)

People with ASPD are early birds: the timing of their sleep–wake cycle is advanced compared to the average population, so they fall asleep too early in the evening to take part in a normal social/family life and wake up too early in the morning.

AMYGDALA

A region of the brain that stores emotionally significant memories of scary and threatening experiences and automatically triggers a stress response whenever it detects a similarity with what's currently going on around you. The amygdala can become inappropriately programmed to produce stress responses when there is no real imminent danger. Retraining the amygdala is possible with hypnotic and NLP techniques.

APNOEA (SLEEP)

With sleep apnoea people periodically stop breathing throughout the night and wake up to catch their breath. Breathing may become interrupted from 10 seconds to over a minute from 5–30 times or more an hour. Sleep apnoea can cause a tremendous strain and should be taken very seriously. Obstructive sleep apnoea is caused by physical collapse of the respiratory airways; it is typically associated with being overweight and radical weight loss should be undertaken as soon as possible once a proper diagnosis has been made; one should also master Buteyko breathing which reduces the likelihood of the airways collapsing. Central sleep apnoea is a problem in the brain with the control of respiration and breathing; unfortunately I have no therapeutic suggestions for this type of sleep apnoea.

BIOLOGICAL CLOCK
See suprachiasmatic nucleus.

BLUE LIGHT
White (normal) light contains a spectrum of colours, all the colours of the rainbow (red, orange, yellow, green, blue, indigo, violet). Only the cyan-green-blue part of the spectrum is detected by the cells in our eyes that tell our biological clock what time of day it is.

BRIGHT LIGHT THERAPY (BLT)
Positioning a very bright light device – ideally predominantly blue light – within one's visual field for 10–20 minutes at a specific time of day to deliberately set the timing of one's biological clock.

BUTEYKO BREATHING
A breathing method that people with anxiety and panic attacks find helpful. It involves letting your breath become shallow, relaxed and minimalistic.

BUTEYKO BREATHING VERSUS PARASYMPATHETIC BREATHING
For a few people performing slow parasympathetic breathing produces a paradoxical effect and actually *increases* levels of stress and anxiety. For these people the very relaxed *minimalistic* Buteyko breathing is the solution; it helps reduce psychological feelings of stress and anxiety and facilitates inducing the relaxation response.

CIRCADIAN RHYTHMS
Circadian rhythms are physical, mental and behavioural changes that follow their roughly 24-hour cycle. These changes are set by signals from our master biological clock called the suprachiasmatic nucleus; exposing the eyes to bright blue light sets the timing of suprachiasmatic nucleus. Circadian rhythms determine the timing of our sleep–wake cycle by

controlling the timing of cortisol production in the morning, and the production of melatonin and falling body temperature in the evening.

CIRCADIAN RHYTHM SLEEP DISORDER (CRSD)

People with circadian rhythm sleep disorders are unable to sleep and wake at the times required to fit in with their normal work, school and social life. This is not insomnia and people with CRSD are generally able to get enough sleep if allowed to sleep and wake at the times dictated by the internal biological clock. Their sleeping time may come on early in the evening and end early in the morning; this is known as advanced sleep phase disorder. Alternatively their natural sleeping time may start and end very late; this is known as delayed sleep phase disorder.

CORTISOL

Cortisol is a hormone released by our adrenal glands. It is released in the morning under the control of our biological clock and whenever we produce a stress response. Over-producing stress responses in the evening prevents cortisol levels from declining and maintains a wakeful state.

DEEP SLEEP

A stage of sleep that we enter into two or three times during the first half of the night. During deep sleep we are the most dissociated from our conscious wakeful state and it is very difficult to wake someone up from this condition. The body's production of growth hormone is at its peak during deep sleep and many important physical repair processes are carried out at this time. When a person is deprived of deep sleep their system will increase the amount of time they spend in deep sleep later on and attempt to recover 100 per cent of the missed deep sleep, which implies adequate deep sleep is vitally important to our well-being. Deep sleep is vulnerable to being disrupted by the presence of excessive stress hormones and alcohol. Cannabis may actually increase the amount of time we spend in deep sleep, however this is at the expense of REM sleep which is important for the mind and memory to work properly.

DELAYED SLEEP PHASE DISORDER (DSPD)

People with DSPD are night owls: the timing of their sleep–wake cycle is delayed compared to the average population so they are still wide awake late into the evening or night long after the average person has fallen asleep and naturally wake up too late in the morning to take part in normal work and daily life. When forced to wake up at what is for them an unnaturally early time people with DSPD regularly suffer from sleep deprivation.

5-HTP

5-hydroxytryptophan naturally occurs in the body and is midway between the amino acid tryptophan and serotonin. Tryptophan is converted into 5-HTP which in turn is converted into the neurotransmitter serotonin, which is then converted into melatonin.

GABA

Gamma-amino butyric acid is the main tranquillising and sedating neurotransmitter in the brain. Without adequate GABA the brain finds it difficult to relax and calm down worrying, anxious and repetitive thoughts. GABA levels can be boosted with GABA supplements and L-theanine.

GHRELIN

Ghrelin is a hormone that has many functions in the body, one of the most significant of which is it strongly influences the brain to feel hungry for specifically high fat and high calorie foods. Simply put ghrelin compels you to eat more calories and ghrelin levels are elevated the day after a bad night's sleep ergo poor sleep can make you gain weight.

INSOMNIA

Insomnia is having problems with falling asleep, staying asleep long enough or both to satisfy your needs for sleep; it may also be sleeping long enough but only achieving very poor quality sleep such that you don't get enough quality sleep and you end up with daytime tiredness. When insomnia lasts for just a few days it is called transient insomnia, when it lasts for several weeks it's called acute insomnia and when it lasts for more than several months it's called chronic insomnia. I recommend if you get acute insomnia you treat it quickly and aggressively throwing every technique in this book at it to prevent it from turning into a chronic insomnia.

INTRINSICALLY PHOTOSENSITIVE RETINAL GANGLION CELLS
See ipRG cells.

IPRG CELLS

The intrinsically photosensitive retinal ganglion cells are specialist cells in our eyes that only respond to blue-cyan coloured light and whose job is to tell the master biological clock when the day starts and this sets the timing of our circadian (daily) physiological cycles, including the timing of our sleep. As long as the ipRG cells continue receiving blue light in the evening including artificial light from TVs, tablets, etc., it prevents melatonin production. When they stop receiving light the suprachiasmatic nucleus (biological clock) tells the pituitary gland to make the sleep hormone melatonin.

JET LAG

Jet lag is a temporary physiological condition where one's circadian rhythm is out of sync with one's current environment. It results from rapid travelling across time zones (travelling East or West) and one's internal biological clock temporarily still being set to one's original starting location; so for example you may now be in New York but your biological clock still thinks it's in London. Many physiological processes are coordinated on a 24-hour clock including the time we sleep, the movement of our digestive system, our peak mental and physical performance, etc. It's possible for jet lag to significantly impact on your performance, if for example you were attending an important meeting when your biological clock was shutting down your mental and physical performance into night-time sleep mode. Using the techniques in this book you can rapidly reset your biological clock and even move it several hours *before* you travel.

LITHINASE

A very low dose highly absorbable form of lithium. This lithium supplement is *not at all* the same as the highly toxic form and dosage of lithium used in psychiatric medicine to treat bipolar syndrome; in fact far from being toxic there is a little evidence that this low dose of lithium has powerful anti-ageing and life extending effects.

MELATONIN

Melatonin is a hormone released into the blood by the pineal gland which in humans induces sleep and sleepiness. Melatonin production is inhibited by light entering the eyes and permitted by darkness. Bright artificial light in the evening can delay and diminish the amount of melatonin we produce and thus how well we sleep; because it's only blue light frequencies that do this we can eliminate this problem by eliminating blue light in our evening environment (see virtual darkness).

Besides its central role in sleep melatonin has other important effects: it is a powerful antioxidant preventing damage to DNA by some cancer-causing carcinogens (see www.the-sleep-solution.com for references). There is growing evidence that the reduced melatonin production that results from artificial evening light increases one's risk of developing cancer, particularly breast cancer. Melatonin may also have important immune boosting effects, anti-ageing effects and reduce the risk of developing Type II diabetes. For more information on the health benefits of this remarkable molecule see the-sleep-solution.com

NEUROTRANSMITTERS
Neurotransmitters are chemical substances that are released at the end of a nerve and transmit the nervous impulse from one nerve cell to another.

OBSTRUCTIVE SLEEP APNOEA
See apnoea.

PARASYMPATHETIC BREATHING TECHNIQUE
Consciously slowing one's breathing down to as little as 2–3 breaths per minute induces a deeply relaxed condition in which the parasympathetic branch of the nervous system becomes dominant and overrides or cancels stress responses in the body.

PARASYMPATHETIC RELAXATION RESPONSE
There is a network of nerves in our body called the autonomic nervous system that runs the level of tension in our body automatically in the background without us having to think about it. There are two opposing sides to the autonomic nervous system: the sympathetic side that when dominant produces stress responses throughout our body and the parasympathetic side which when dominant produces relaxation and switches off stress responses throughout our body. The parasympathetic nervous system is said to be outside our conscious control; however, if we systematically relax the muscles throughout our body, slow or relax our breathing and make our mind go passive we can activate the parasympathetic nervous system and initiate the relaxation response.

REM SLEEP

Rapid eye movement or REM sleep is a distinct phase of sleep which occurs mainly in the second half of the night. During REM sleep we do most of our dreaming and consolidate the things we have learned during the day into our long-term memory, therefore it is important to get enough REM sleep to study and learn new things. The name rapid eye movement comes from the fact that during the sleep phase our eyes move rapidly from side to side when we are dreaming.

RESTLESS LEGS SYNDROME

Restless legs syndrome causes sudden urges to relieve aches and pains in the legs by moving or rubbing them; the sudden movements are sufficient to wake one up or prevent one falling asleep therefore causing insomnia.

SLEEP DEBT

If the number of hours you're actually sleeping is less than the number of hours your individual body needs to sleep you build up a sleep debt. Just a few minutes less sleep than we need every night can surreptitiously build up a sleep debt. It's a popular myth that you can build up a bit of a sleep debt during the week and then properly pay it all back at the weekend by sleeping longer; although it is true that the brain will extend the length of time you spend in deep sleep to recover lost deep sleep, we do not fully recover our REM sleep which we need for healthy mental functioning and suffer diminished mental performance every day we have sleep debt. Sleep debt looks different to chronic fatigue; you could find the signs to look out for to indicate you have sleep debt elsewhere in the book (see page 48).

SLEEP–WAKE CYCLE

The roughly 24-hour cycle of sleeping and waking that is part of healthy daily physiology. It is run primarily under the control of our master biological clock the suprachiasmatic nucleus, the timing of which is set most significantly by exposure to bright light in the morning.

SEROTONIN

Serotonin is a calming and inhibiting chemical in the brain, a so-called neurotransmitter. Low levels of serotonin are associated with some types of depression; see my website (www.balancingbrainchemistry.co.uk) for more on this. When our suprachiasmatic nucleus detects the lights have gone out, either because all the lights are off or because we have put ourselves into virtual darkness, our pineal gland starts to produce melatonin from serotonin; in fact the levels of serotonin in the brain plummet as it is used up to make melatonin.

For good sleep we need adequate levels of serotonin to make adequate levels of melatonin.

SUBCONSCIOUS REPROGRAMMING

Our subconscious can learn how to do even quite complex tasks like driving a car; it can also be taught associations like your bed is a place you easily fall asleep in. However, the subconscious can be taught unhelpful things like bad driving habits or to associate your bed with insomnia and not falling asleep. The unconscious learns how to do things through repetitive actions and unhelpful learning conditioned into the subconscious can be reprogrammed and unlearned by repeating the correct, helpful behaviour we want and through hypnotically talking to the subconscious.

SUPRACHIASMATIC NUCLEUS

The suprachiasmatic nucleus (SCN) is our body's master internal biological clock; it is a remarkable tiny bundle of nerves in the brain with inbuilt rhythmic, timekeeping properties. The SCN sends out signals at specific times of day to different body systems such as the adrenal glands, the digestive system, and practically every aspect of our sleep system such as our core temperature and melatonin production, etc. The SCN runs the timing of many aspects of our physiology, so when the timing of the SCN is out of sync with the eating and sleeping schedule we are living we can feel jetlagged and terrible. The timing of the SCN can be reset on a daily basis by exposing the eyes to bright blue light; we can use this to treat circadian rhythm sleep disorders and even pre-empt jet lag.

TOTAL DARKNESS

Sleeping in a totally dark bedroom prevents stray light from outside the room and light sources within the room reducing melatonin production; the more melatonin you produce, the better your sleep. The biological clock in people with ASPD (early birds) may be supersensitive to dawn light entering their sleeping area and be woken up by it; sleeping in total darkness is an important technique in overcoming this unpleasant condition.

TRYPTOPHAN

Tryptophan is a naturally occurring amino acid (building blocks of proteins) present in all protein-containing foods. Tryptophan is converted into the calming neurotransmitter serotonin which is subsequently converted into melatonin. When naturally consumed in protein foods tryptophan can be pushed out of the way by the other amino acids and may not readily pass through the blood brain barrier. Supplementing tryptophan on its own last thing at night removes the competition posed by other amino acids enabling it to flow more freely into the brain providing us with more of the building blocks needed to make the serotonin and melatonin needed for good sleep. Tryptophan is safe and nonaddictive; however, it should not be supplemented at the same time as taking SSRI antidepressant drugs. On my insomnia cure I use tryptophan as a sleep aid to kick-start better sleeping and or assist withdrawal from sleeping pills.

VIRTUAL DARKNESS

Our biological clock only uses blue light to register the presence of daylight and eliminating blue frequencies of light by wearing amber glasses or using yellow light bulbs effectively sends the biological clock into total darkness; however, we can still see our way around because our eyes can detect other colours of light. This low blue light environment is called virtual darkness and it is useful because it enables us to live with artificial lighting while extending the period of time that our biological clock spends in darkness which increases the length of time we produce melatonin which helps us sleep and fights cancer.

References

Allen, R. (2004) 'Dopamine and iron in the pathophysiology of restless legs syndrome (RLS).' *Sleep Medicine 5*, 4, 385–391.

Allen, R. P. and Earley C. J. (2007) 'The role of iron in restless legs syndrome.' *Movement Disorders 22, Suppl. 18*, S440–448.

Anthony, C. and Anthony, W. (1999) *The Art of Napping at Work.* New York: Larson Publications.

Blask, D. E. (2009) 'Melatonin, sleep disturbance and cancer risk.' *Sleep Medicine Reviews 13*, 4, 257–264.

Blumenfeld, A. J., Fleshmer, N., Casselman, B. and Trachtenberg, J. (2000) 'Nutritional aspects of prostate cancer: a review.' *Canadian Journal of Urology 7*, 1, 927–935.

Buck, A. C., Cox, R., Rees, R. W., Ebeling, L. and John, A. (1990) 'Treatment of outflow tract obstruction due to benign prostatic hyperplasia with the pollen extract, cernilton. A double-blind, placebo-controlled study.' *British Journal of Urology 66*, 4, 398–404.

Clark, L. C., Dalkin, B., Krongrad, A., Combs. G. F. Jr. *et al.* (1998) 'Decreased incidence of prostate cancer with selenium supplementation: results of a double-blind cancer prevention trial.' *British Journal of Urology 81*, 5, 730–734.

Clarke, R., Smith, A. D., Jobst, K. A., Refsum, H., Sutton, L. and Ueland, P. M. (1998) 'Folate, vitamin B12, and serum total homocysteine levels in confirmed Alzheimer disease.' *Archives of Neurology 55*, 11, 1449–1455.

Feychting, M., Osterlund, B. and Ahlbom, A. (1998) 'Reduced cancer incidence among the blind.' *Epidemiology 9*, 5, 490–494.

Ficca, G., Axelsson, J., Mollicone, D. J., Muto, V. and Vitiello, M. V. (2010) 'Naps, cognition and performance.' *Sleep Medicine Reviews 14*, 4, 249–258.

Flynn-Evans, E. E., Stevens, R. G., Tabandeh, H., Schernhammer, E. S. and Lockley, S. W. (2009) 'Total visual blindness is protective against breast cancer.' *Cancer Causes Control 20*, 9, 1753–1756.

Gałuszko-Węgielnik, M., Jakuszkowiak-Wojten, K., Wiglusz, M. S., Cubała, W. J. and Landowski, J. (2012) 'The efficacy of Cognitive-Behavioural Therapy (CBT) as related to sleep quality and hyperarousal level in the treatment of primary insomnia.' *Psychiatria Danubia 24*, Suppl. 1, S51–55.

Gooley, J. J., Chamberlain, K., Smith, K. A., Rajaratnam, S. M. *et al.* (2011) 'Exposure to room light before bedtime suppresses melatonin onset and shortens melatonin duration in humans.' *Journal of Clinical Endocrinology and Metabolism 96*, 3, E463–E472.

Hahn, R. A. (1991) 'Profound bilateral blindness and the incidence of breast cancer.' *Epidemiology 2*, 3, 208–210.

Hansen, J. (2001) 'Light at night, shiftwork, and breast cancer risk.' JNCI: *Journal of the National Cancer Institute 93*, 20, 1513–1515.

Hansler, R. L. (2008). *Great Sleep! Reduced Cancer!: A Scientific Approach to Great Sleep and Reduced Risk of Cancer*. Charleston, SC: BookSurge.

Hauri, P. J. (1997) 'Can we mix behavioral therapy with hypnotics when treating insomniacs?' *Sleep: Journal of Sleep Research & Sleep Medicine 20*, 12, 1111–1118.

Honma, K., Kohsaka, M., Fukuda, N., Morita, N. and Honma, S. (1992) 'Effects of vitamin B12 on plasma melatonin rhythm in humans: Increased light sensitivity phase-advances the circadian clock?' *Experientia 48*, 8, 716–720.

Horne, J. A. and Staff, L. H. (1983) 'Exercise and sleep: Body-heating effects.' *Sleep 6*, 1, 36–46.

Huang, T., Chen, Y., Yang, B., Yang, J., Wahlqvist, M. L. and Li, D. (2012) 'Meta-analysis of B vitamin supplementation on plasma homocysteine, cardiovascular and all-cause mortality.' *Clinical Nutrition 31*, 4, 448–454.

Itsipoulos, C. Hodge, A. and Kaimakamis, M. (2009) 'Can the Mediterranean diet prevent prostate cancer?' *Molecular Nutrition & Food Research (Special Issue: Diet and Prostate Cancer) 53*, 2, 227–239.

Jacobs, G. D., Pace-Schott, E. F., Stickgold, R. and Otto, M. W. (2004) 'Cognitive behavior therapy and pharmacotherapy for insomnia: a randomized controlled trial and direct comparison.' *Archives of Internal Medicine 164*, 17, 1888–1896.

Kripke, D. F. *The Dark Side of Sleeping Pills: Mortality and Cancer Risks, Which Pills to Avoid & Better Alternatives*. Available at www.darksideofsleepingpills.com/pdf/darkside.pdf, accessed on 3 June 2013.

Kripke, D. F., Juarez, S., Cole, R. J. and Ancoli-Israel, S. et al. (1994) 'Adult Illumination Exposures and Some Correlations with Symptoms.' In T. Hiroshige and K. Honma (eds) *Evolution of Circadian Clock*. Sapporo: Hokkaido University Press, 349–360.

Kripke, D. F., Langer, R. D. and Kline, L. E. (2012) 'Hypnotics' association with mortality or cancer: a matched cohort study.' *BMJ Open*, 2:e000850, doi:10.1136/bmjopen-2012-000850.

Kristal, A. R., Stanford, J. L., Cohen, J. H., Wicklund, K. and Patterson, R. E. (1999) 'Vitamin and mineral supplement use is associated with reduced risk of prostate cancer.' *Cancer Epidemiology, Biomarkers & Prevention 8*, 887–892.

Kukala *et al.* (1999) in Hansler, R.L. (2008) *Great Sleep! Reduced Cancer! A scientific Approach to Great Sleep and Reduced Cancer Risk*. Available at www.bluelights.com.

Lin, H.-H., Tsai, P.-S., Fang, S.C. and Liu, J.-F. (2011) 'Effect of kiwifruit consumption on sleep quality in adults with sleep problems.' *Asia Pacific Journal of Clinical Nutrition 20*, 2, 169–174.

Morin, C. M., Bootzin, R. R., Buysse, D. J., Edinger, J. D., Espie, C. A. and Lichstein, K. L. (2006) 'Psychological and behavioural treatment of insomnia: update of the recent evidence (1998–2004).' *Sleep 29*, 11, 1398–1414.

Naska, A., Oikonomou, E., Trichopoulou, A., Psaltopoulou, T. and Trichopoulos, D. (2007) 'Siesta in healthy adults and coronary mortality in the general population.' *Archives of Internal Medicine 167*, 296–301.

Okawa, M., Takahashi, K., Egashira, K., Furuta, H. *et al.* (1997) 'Vitamin B12 treatment for delayed sleep phase syndrome: A multi-center double-blind study.' *Psychiatry and Clinical Neurosciences 51*, 5, 275–279.

Passos, G. S., Poyares, D., Santana, M. G., Garbuio, S. A., Tufik, S. and Mello, M. T. (2010) 'Effect of acute physical exercise on patients with chronic primary insomnia.' *Journal of Clinical Sleep Medicine 6*, 3, 250–275.

Pollard, M. and Wolter, W. (2000) 'Prevention of spontaneous prostate-related cancer in Lobund-Wistar rats by a soy protein isolate/isoflavone diet.' *Prostate (Special Issue: Festschrift in Honor of Dr. Gerald P. Murphy) 45*, 2, 101–105.

Reiter, R. J., Tan, D. X., Korkmaz. A., Erren, T.C. *et al.* (2007) 'Light at night, chronodisruption, melatonin suppression, and cancer risk: a review.' *Critical Reviews in Oncogenesis 13*, 4, 303–328.

Rosekind, M. R., Smith, R. M., Miller, D. L., Co, E. L. *et al.* (1995) 'Alertness management: strategic naps in operational settings.' *Journal of Sleep Research 4*, Suppl. s2, 62–66.

Rupp, T. L., Wesensten, N. J., Bliese, P. D. and Balkin, T. J. (2009) 'Banking sleep: Realization of benefits during subsequent sleep restriction and recovery.' *Sleep 32*, 3, 311–321.

ScienceDaily (2008) 'Office workers given blue light to help alertness.' Available at www.sciencedaily.com/releases/2008/10/081029105807.htm, accessed on 3 June 2013.

ScienceDaily (2010) 'Lack of morning light keeping teenagers up at night.' Available at www.sciencedaily.com/releases/2010/02/100216140305.htm, accessed on 3 June 2013.

ScienceDaily (2007) 'Chronically sleep deprived? You can make up for lost sleep.' Available at www.sciencedaily.com/releases/2007/07/070702145153.htm, accessed on 23 April.

Seligman, M. (1998) Learned Optimism. New York: Pocket Books.

Smith, A. D., Smith, S. M., de Jager, C. A. and Whitbread, P. 'Homocysteine-lowering by B vitamins slows the rate of brain atrophy in mild cognitive impairment: a randomized trial.' PLoS One 5, 9, 12244.

Stevens, R. G. (2009) 'Artificial lighting in the industrialized world: circadian disruption and breast cancer.' Cancer Causes & Control 17, 4, 501–507.

Roughey, C., Aggarwal, N., Li, H. and Wilson, R. et al. (2011) 'Vitamin B12, cognition, and brain MRI measures: A cross-sectional examination.' Neurology 77, 13, 1276–1282.

Tomoda, A., Miike, T., Uezono, K. and Kawasaki, T. (1994) 'A school refusal case with biological rhythm disturbance and melatonin therapy.' Brain and Development 16, 1, 71–76.

Wahnschaffe, A., Haedel, S., Rodenbeck, A., Stoll, C. et al. (2013) 'Out of the lab and into the bathroom: evening short-term exposure to conventional light suppresses melatonin and increases alertness perception.' International Journal of Molecular Sciences 14, 1, 2573–2589.

Wood, B., Rea, M. S., Plitnick, B. and Figueiro, M. G. (2013) 'Light level and duration of exposure determine the impact of self-luminous tablets on melatonin suppression.' Applied Ergonomics 44, 2, 237–240.

Wurtman, R. J. and Fernstrom, J. D. (1975) 'Control of brain monoamine synthesis by diet and plasma amino acids.' American Journal of Clinical Nutrition 28, 6, 638–647.

Wurtman, R. J., Wurtman, J. J., Regan, M. M., McDermott, J. M. et al. (2003) 'Effects of normal meals rich in carbohydrates or proteins on plasma tryptophan and tyrosine ratios.' American Journal of Clinical Nutrition 77, 1, 128–132.

Wyatt, R. J., Kupfer, D. J., Sjoerdsma, A., Engelman, K., Fram, D. H. and Snyder, F. (1970) 'Effects of L-tryptophan (a natural sedative) on human sleep.' The Lancet 296, 7678, 842–846.

Yakut, M., Ustün, Y., Kabaçam, G. and Soykan, I. (2010) 'Serum vitamin B12 and folate status in patients with inflammatory bowel diseases.' European Journal of Internal Medicine 21, 4, 320–323.

Further Reading

American Academy of Sleep Medicine (2008) 'Bright light therapy may improve nocturnal sleep in mothers.' Available at www.aasmnet.org/articles.aspx?id=878, accessed on 3 June 2013.

American Academy of Sleep Medicine (2010) 'Bright light therapy improves sleep disturbances in soldiers with combat PTSD.' Available at www.aasmnet.org/articles.aspx?id=1719, accessed on 3 June 2013.

Figueiro, M. G. and Rea, M. S. (2010) 'Evening daylight may cause adolescents to sleep less in spring than in winter.' *Chronobiology International 27*, 6, 1242–1258.

Figueiro, M. G. and Rea, M. S. (2012) 'Short-wavelength light enhances cortisol awakening response in sleep-restricted adolescents.' *International Journal of Endocrinology.* Available at www.hindawi.com/journals/ije/2012/301935/, accessed on 3 June 2013.

Figueiro, M. G., Bierman, A., Plitnick, B. and Rea, M. S. (2009) 'Preliminary evidence that both blue and red light can induce alertness at night.' *BMC Neuroscience 10*, 105.

Hartmann, E. (1974) 'L-tryptophan: A possible natural hypnotic substance.' *Journal of the American Medical Association 230*, 12, 1680–1681.

Kloog, I., Stevens, R. G., Haim, A. and Portnov, B. A. (2010) 'Night-time light level co-distributes with breast cancer incidence worldwide.' *Cancer Causes and Control 21*, 12, 2059–2066.

Kripke, D. F. *Brighten Your Life: How Bright Light Therapy Helps with Low Mood, Sleep Problems and Jet Lag.* Available at www.brightenyourlife.info/, accessed on 3 June 2013.

Spivey, A. (2010) 'Light pollution: Light at night and breast cancer risk worldwide.' *Environmental Health Perspectives 118*, 12.

Turner, P. L., Van Someren, E. J. and Mainster, M. A. (2010) 'The role of environmental light in sleep and health: Effects of ocular aging and cataract surgery.' *Sleep Medicine Review 14*, 4, 269–280.

Contact Details and Getting the Free Recordings

To receive the digital recordings to accompany this book simply send me an e-mail asking for the sleep better recordings. My address is: sleep@the-sleep-solution.com.

N.B. The recordings are large files and may need to be sent one at a time.

For more information on sleeping better and the techniques in this book, see my website: www.the-sleep-solution.com.

For more information on neurotransmitters and treating depression, bipolar syndrome and anxiety with natural remedies, see: www.balancingbrainchemistry.co.uk.

For more information on healthy diet, how to detoxify, weight-loss and naturopathic medicine, see: www. PeterSmithUK.com.

Index